A Computational Approach to Statistical Arguments in Ecology and Evolution

Scientists need statistics. Increasingly this is accomplished using computational approaches. Freeing readers from the constraints, mysterious formulas, and sophisticated mathematics of classical statistics, this book is ideal for researchers who want to take control of their own statistical arguments.

It demonstrates how to use spreadsheet macros to calculate the probability distribution predicted for any statistic by any hypothesis. This enables readers to use anything that can be calculated (or observed) from their data as a test statistic, and hypothesize any probabilistic mechanism that can generate data sets similar in structure to the one observed.

A wide range of natural examples drawn from ecology, evolution, anthropology, paleontology, and related fields give valuable insights into the application of the described techniques, while complete example macros and useful procedures demonstrate the methods in action and provide starting points for readers to use or modify in their own research.

George F. Estabrook is a Professor of Botany in the Department of Ecology and Evolutionary Biology at the University of Michigan, Ann Arbor. He is interested in the application of mathematics and computing to biology, and has taught graduate courses on the subject for more than 30 years.

A Computational Approach to Statistical Arguments in Ecology and Evolution

GEORGE F. ESTABROOK

University of Michigan, Ann Arbor

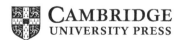 CAMBRIDGE
UNIVERSITY PRESS

CAMBRIDGE
UNIVERSITY PRESS

University Printing House, Cambridge CB2 8BS, United Kingdom

One Liberty Plaza, 20th Floor, New York, NY 10006, USA

477 Williamstown Road, Port Melbourne, VIC 3207, Australia

314-321, 3rd Floor, Plot 3, Splendor Forum, Jasola District Centre, New Delhi - 110025, India

103 Penang Road, #05-06/07, Visioncrest Commercial, Singapore 238467

Cambridge University Press is part of the University of Cambridge.

It furthers the University's mission by disseminating knowledge in the pursuit of education, learning and research at the highest international levels of excellence.

www.cambridge.org
Information on this title: www.cambridge.org/9781107004306

First published 2011

A catalogue record for this publication is available from the British Library

ISBN 978-1-107-00430-6 Hardback

Additional resources for this publication at www.cambridge.org/9781107004306

Contents

Acknowledgments

In the mid 1980s, Neal Oden quit his boring job as a computer programmer and joined the Ph.D. program of the Department of Biology at the University of Michigan to become my eighth Ph.D. student. Neal had read a journal article in which the authors claimed that when data sampled a given probability distribution, the predicted distribution of a statistic they had invented would asymptotically converge to a known pre-calculated distribution of classical statistics. From the authors' explanation, it was not clear to Neal why. So he wrote a computer program that used a random number generator to sample the given distribution to create a large data set, and calculate the statistic; his program repeated this 1000 times to estimate the predicted distribution. The middle 80% was pretty close to the classical distribution, but upper and lower 10% differed. By doing this, Neal showed me how easy it is to make accurate estimations of the probability distribution for any statistic predicted by any hypothesis of random. Thank you, Neal. I began to apply Neal's idea in collaboration with other colleagues, and eventually offered a course to graduate students.

The many students who took my course, BIO 480 and later EEB 480, have contributed much to the development of this book, which has gone through a half dozen unpublished editions over the past decade in response to their helpful suggestions and requests.

One of the major stumbling blocks for students trying to use these concepts and techniques has been the need to learn enough computer programming to implement them. I taught my course originally using PASCAL, a programming language designed explicitly to teach students good programming practices. Even with PASCAL, the INPUT, OUTPUT, and MEMORY MANAGEMENT details were especially challenging for students who had never programmed before. A few years ago, my 18th Ph.D. student, Don Schoolmaster, showed me how to program spreadsheet macros that read from, and write to, spreadsheets. This eliminates problems with INPUT, OUTPUT, and MEMORY MANAGEMENT, which makes the programming much more accessible to students. Virtually all students are familiar with spreadsheets, even if they have never programmed a macro. Thank you, Don.

Keith Hunley, a former EEB 480 student and now a professor at the University of New Mexico, read much of the pre-final draft of the book. He made hundreds of suggestions that improved the clarity and organization. Thank you, Keith.

My wife, Virginia Hutton Estabrook Ph.D., helped me with drawing the figures, organizing the literature cited, and grappling with the WINDOWS operating system. She also read some of the pre-final draft and made helpful suggestions. Thank you, Virginia.

1 | Introduction

1.1 About the book

Purpose

The purpose of this book is to teach you how to make statistical arguments using computational approaches. Such arguments are based on test-statistic probability distributions predicted by hypotheses, as in the classical approach. Unlike the classical approach, these predicted probability distributions are calculated by direct simulation of the hypotheses themselves. This approach enables you to use anything that can be calculated (or observed) from your data as a test statistic, and hypothesize any probabilistic mechanism that can generate data sets similar in structure to the one you observed. This approach frees you from the constraints, mysterious formulas, and sophisticated mathematics that classical statistics entails, and enables you to take personal control of your statistical arguments. To access this power, you will need to learn to program a computer (if you do not already know how). This task is greatly simplified through the use of spreadsheet macros, which enable the organization and input of data, as well as the output of results, using the spreadsheet itself. Many of you are already familiar with spreadsheets. The macros you will need to program will serve mostly to perform calculations, so that you will need to learn only a small sub-set of the programming language. In this book, I discuss basic hypothesis-testing statistical argument, data structures, choice of test statistics, some probability theory and its use in formulating hypotheses, and enough programming techniques to specify the calculations that simulate data sets using probabilistic hypotheses. Much of the discourse is with natural examples. Although this computational approach to statistical argument is widely applicable, these examples are mostly drawn from anthropology, ecology, evolution, and paleontology, which are my areas of interest, and those of most of my students.

Intended readers

This book is intended for readers who aspire to become, are already becoming, or who have become, research scientists who would like to feel more in control of their statistical arguments. It does not expect you to have prior training in statistics or computer programming, but some of my students who have had such training found this book valuable because it provided a very different view of these subjects, especially of statistics. Earlier versions of this book have existed in unpublished form for the past decade. I used them to teach my course on computational approaches to statistical argument at the University of Michigan. My students have been mostly Ph.D. students (about half in biological anthropology, and the others in paleontology, ecology, and evolution, with a few other areas occasionally represented). However, a few masters students, undergraduates planning to attend graduate school, post-doctoral fellows, and even fellow faculty have also participated.

Spreadsheets – This book will teach you how to make statistical arguments using a computational approach. To access this power, this text will show you all you need to know to program macros for an EXCEL spreadsheet. Here you will find examples of complete EXCEL macros. You can cut and paste them into your own EXCEL workbook and run them there. However, to do just this would miss the point. These examples show you how to program specific tasks, and are intended to be part of your personal programming manual, together with the more general explanations in the text. After all, you are reading this text because you want to free yourself from dependency on canned programs, stat packages, etc., to take responsibility for your own statistical arguments. Many students find it effective to copy examples into their macro editor using their keyboard, and then experiment with modifications of them to solidify their understanding. Later, when programming macros for your own research applications, you will be able to re-use blocks of statements from these examples.

Some of my students, who felt anxious at the beginning of my course because they did not already know how to program, bought books about programming, or downloaded things from the web about programming, or got help from a friend who had taken a course on programming. Because this book presents only a small fraction of the macro programming language, there is less to learn; extra, unnecessary information leads to confusion and delay. This book has all you need to know to do the things you need to do to start taking a computational approach to statistical argument using a spreadsheet. A few of my students, after they had mastered the concepts of this book, decided that they wanted to climb the steep learning curve to master an object-oriented, general programming language, such as JAVA. This enabled them to participate more fully in the present-day world of computing, but did not enhance their ability to take a computational approach to statistical arguments.

Why use computation

Over the past decade, the use of computational approaches to statistical argument in research publications has increased, although it is still not widely used, because, in part, many scientists lack the ability to access these techniques, and those who can mostly include those who are also very well grounded in the techniques of classical statistics. As a consequence, such computational approaches are often seen as especially sophisticated, when in fact they are much easier to master than a strong grounding in classical statistics. Many early career scientists remain unable to access computational approaches to statistical argument mostly because there is no effective, entry-level instructional book to teach them. This is such a book.

This book describes methods for formulating hypotheses and for calculating predictions from them so that they may be tested with data. These methods enable you to formulate hypotheses and to design experiments, so that you can make inferences from data, free of the burden of unwanted mathematical assumptions. Until recently, few natural scientists who wanted to reason with quantitative data could do so with a full understanding of the data analytic methods they were expected to use. Why? During the early part of the twentieth century, the inventors of statistics made assumptions and used mathematical techniques in order to avoid the impossibly large amounts of computation that would otherwise have been required. They brought a new level of rigor to inference making, which made a major contribution to the methods of natural scientists and other scholars. However, this (now) classical approach to statistics presents three problems: (1) the mathematics is too hard for most otherwise excellent research scientists to master; (2) the assumptions were NOT what scientists needed to include in their hypotheses; and (3) as a consequence of the inaccessibility of the mathematics and the irrelevance of the assumptions, many scientists turned to a statistical expert to decide the details of forming a hypothesis and choosing a test statistic, and did not take direct responsibility for their own hypotheses and arguments.

Now, with personal computers, you can do vast quantities of calculations rapidly and painlessly. So claim power over, and responsibility for, your own statistical arguments. This book will help students (undergraduate, graduate, or established professionals) who aspire to careers that include the practice of scientific research (experimental and/or comparative) to learn how to structure data to facilitate questions, to hypothesize probabilistic mechanisms that describe variability, to choose relevant test statistics, and to instruct personal computers to put those mechanisms into motion to simulate the probability distribution predicted by their hypothesis for that statistic.

Prerequisites

Although the examples here will come primarily from biological and cultural anthropology, paleontology, ecology, and organismal evolution, the methods and concepts are more generally applicable. In addition to a strong desire to take responsibility for your own hypotheses and arguments, you should also have a (nearly) complete undergraduate major in a science, broadly construed, to be able to take full advantage of this book. A background in organismal natural science (e.g., ecology, evolution, biological anthropology, paleontology, archeology, natural resources, botany, among others) will help you recognize the examples in this book, but any social or natural science background is sufficient. Some recollection of high-school algebra will also be useful.

How to use this book

The book starts with a description of some basic principles, and programming concepts. It then uses a published case study to show you in more detail how to instruct your personal computer to carry out the computation you need to put these principles into practice. These pages are intended to give you an initial feel for this approach. Please do not expect to understand or remember every concept on your first reading. These concepts and techniques will be visited repeatedly through the rest of the book. When you have had a little practice programming spreadsheet macros yourself, come back and read these pages again. Data structures and probability mechanisms will continue to be described so that you can calculate predictions using your personal computer. You will be shown specific programming techniques, with examples using spreadsheet macros ready for you to use as examples and modify to meet your own needs. These computational methods avoid the need to understand the mathematics, and to accept the pre-determined assumptions and test statistics of classical statistics. They enable you to understand every step of your own argument.

Although any of several computer source languages could have been used for these instructional purposes, I chose EXCEL macros. There are many good reasons for this choice. EXCEL macros are programmed in a so-called structured language, which means that data structures are explicit and instructions are hierarchically nested to reflect the logic of the algorithms. Most of you are at least somewhat familiar with spreadsheets already, even if you have never programmed macros for them. Much of what is difficult about programming in a more general language, such as PASCAL\DELPHI, C or JAVA, is managing the input of data and the output of results (so called I/O), especially when graphics interfaces (like WINDOWS and MAC operating systems) are involved. Spreadsheet macros can read data right from a spreadsheet, and can write results to a spreadsheet as well. Thus, most of the programming you will need to learn will be to instruct the computer to carry out the calculations you want it to perform. With less concern for I/O, it is much easier to learn enough about programming so that you can write spreadsheet macros to carry out the computational approach to statistical argument described here.

To get the most out of this book, it is a very good idea to copy, using your keyboard, the example programs (macros) in the text into your spreadsheet macro editor and run them yourself. Once you get started, you can experiment with your own modifications of them, and later the text will challenge you with solving problems by writing your own programs, which you will be able to do by copying from the examples you already have. To do this you will need access to a personal computer that runs a spreadsheet that enables you to write macros. Microsoft chose to remove macro programming entirely from EXCEL 2008 for MACs, and to obscure access to it in

EXCEL 2007 for WINDOWS. To take advantage of macros in EXCEL on a Mac you will need the 2004 (or earlier) version. Macro programming is readily available in earlier versions of EXCEL: (1) open EXCEL, (2) bring down the "Tools" menu, (3) open the "macros" sub-menu and (4) click on "Visual Basic Editor". The macros hiding place in EXCEL 2007 for WINDOWS is found like this: (1) open EXCEL, (2) click the "office" button in the upper left, which opens a little window where in the bottom right you can (3) click a button called "EXCEL options", which opens a menu where you can (4) click "Show developer tab" and then "OK", which closes all these little windows and leaves EXCEL open with the developer tab showing, where you can now (5) click "Visual Basic". Later, when you start programming yourself, how to use the macro editor and run macros will be explained in more detail.

To take a computational approach to statistical argument you will need to be able to instruct a computer to perform computation. However, this text is mostly not about computer programming; it is about statistical arguments, and how to make them using computation, instead of classical statistics. Toward this goal, I will discuss the nature of statistical argument, data structures, the choice of test statistics, and probability concepts. To do this, the text will rely heavily on examples, mostly taken from real questions asked by real scientists, using real data from the natural world, or using simplified data to make the calculations easier, while illustrating the concepts more clearly.

Brief overview

A discussion of argument styles places scientific statistical argument in context with other argument styles common in our culture. Scientific argument is based on hypothesis, prediction, and comparison with data. There are four parts: (1) intellectual foundation enables a question and disciplines observations; (2) data structure enables a statistical hypothesis; (3) probability concepts are part of a statistical hypothesis; and (4) a test statistic is a way to calculate something relevant from your data. A statistical hypothesis predicts a probability distribution for the text statistic.

You can calculate the value of any statistic from your data set. You can also calculate the probability distribution for that statistic predicted by any hypothesis that includes a random process capable of generating data sets with the same structure. To do this, you write a program for your computer. To use computation to make statistical scientific arguments, you need only a few programming concepts. These few concepts are described in the context of natural examples, using spreadsheet macros. Some history of programming concepts is followed by explicit description of the concepts and language of EXCEL, the macro programming that you need to take a computational approach to statistical argument. Now you can start programming yourself, with explicit instructions to use the EXCEL macro editor.

The first example is about a plant adaptation. It integrates scientific argument with the steps you can take to write an EXCEL spreadsheet macro to calculate for a test statistic the probability distribution predicted for it by a hypothesis. Sub CARPEL presents all the programming statements of the complete macro that implements this example. However, your practice is the essential step toward being able to use the concepts and methods of this book in your own research. Next you can follow specific instructions for how to practice. An easy, but realistic, problem is posed and then solved step by step, with advice for effective programming.

The importance of choosing a relevant test statistic is discussed in the context of a specific example taken from paleontology. This example is continued to show you how to create a macro to calculate the realized significance of a relevant test statistic. Sub PERIOD presents all the programming statements of the complete macro that implements this example, and some new programming techniques are introduced.

Next, random variables and their distributions are described somewhat more formally. You are shown how spreadsheet macros use a random number generator to create and plot probability distributions, so that you can see what they look like. Arithmetic with random variables is not the same as arithmetic with numbers. You are shown how to think about and do arithmetic with random variables, using a computational approach. Expected value and variance are properties of a probability distribution that can be useful in your scientific arguments. You are shown how to write macros to estimate expected value and variance.

Another technique for hypothesizing a probability mechanism is called re-sampling data. In the context of a natural example, an unusual but appropriate test statistic is described, and you are shown how to calculate the probability distribution predicted for it by the hypothesis of re-sampling data. Procedures are macros inside a main macro. They enable blocks of instructions to be executed in more than one place in a main macro, without copying them again. This is illustrated using the example of the shell sort. The SORT and PERMUTE procedures are used to illustrate some concepts of testing procedures to increase confidence that they are working properly before they are called by other macros.

The concept of a family of parametric distributions is introduced with the binomial distributions. A formula to calculate probabilities for distributions in the Poisson family is derived in the context of spatial distribution of trees in a savanna. Programming techniques to sample a Poisson distribution are presented. The family of normal distributions is the limiting sum of many independent samples of any random variable. A macro to sample a normal distribution is described. The negative binomial, chi square, and F distributions are briefly described. Later in the context of goodness-of-fit, chi square will be discussed in more detail. A macro to calculate the percentiles of any distribution is described.

The family of data structures, called a linear model, is a useful concept from classical statistics. There is a variety of ways to quantify the error made by a variety of ways to summarize data. The classical way to choose a linear model family member to summarize your data is to minimize squared error. Techniques to discover a particular linear model that minimizes the squared error in summarizing your data are explained. Matrix notation is introduced to describe the calculating formulas that emerge from this explanation. Natural examples use simplified data to better illustrate concepts. One application of a linear model determines a line that minimizes squared error, while summarizing the relationship between two different measurements of the same things. The concepts are presented in the context of a natural example, and a procedure to implement this application is described. A linear model is a way to structure and describe data. It specifies no hypothesized random process to generate data, and no test statistics. To hypothesize a random process, the computational approaches of re-sampling and permutation depart from classical statistics. A computational approach enables the use of any test statistic. A macro to test the significance of the sum of squared errors is described as an example. The concepts of two-way analysis of variance are illustrated using natural examples from ecology, and a procedure for inverting matrices is described.

An estimator is a random variable used to estimate a parameter of the distribution of some other random variable. An estimator is created by doing arithmetic with observed data, hypothesized to be sampling a member of a family of parametric distributions. Consistent, unbiased, and maximum likelihood properties of estimators are explained. Do samples of an unknown random variable (your data) seem to be sampling a given random variable? One way to answer using the classical chi square statistic is discussed in some detail. Computational techniques to compute its predicted probability distribution are presented. With these techniques any relevant statistic can be used; alternative statistics are described.

What can happen when two random processes both participate in generating data? In the artificial example here, you can test a simpler hypothesis to distinguish how two random processes interact. Macro programming techniques are shown. Subtler concerns for choice of test statistic are examined. Finally, a natural example is discussed. Random walks, more general auto-regressive series, and Markov chains, are described, with natural examples.

A computational approach to the analysis of covariance is illustrated with an example of the coevolution of two properties of the same species over time, and a macro to implement this approach. Statistical tests for difference in sexual dimorphism between two species of different size are confounded by size difference. Re-scaling techniques to address this kind of problem are described. Sub SEXDIMO presents the programming statements that implement this example.

How can you get away with peeking at data? Usually, arguments based on classical statistics are less valid if you look at data before you formulate a hypothesis that you intend to test with them. Natural examples illustrate ways to incorporate into the hypothesis the peeking itself. Using a computational approach, you can calculate valid predicted probability distributions for test statistics, even if you peeked.

Two different ways to classify the same collection of entities can be related or independent. The classical approach to testing this independence statistically is problematic with small amounts of data. A computational approach can help. ACTUS2, "Analysis of Contingency Tables Using Simulation, version 2" is an example of a computational approach to statistical argument that I have published. ACTUS2 is a program that uses computation to test for dependencies in sparse contingency tables. How to interpret the results of ACTUS2 is described. Spreadsheet ACTUS is a macro that implements the two hypotheses of independence of ACTUS2, using a spreadsheet for input and output. This section explains how to use it, with explicit instructions. Sub ACTUS presents all the programming statements of the complete macro that implements spreadsheet ACTUS.

1.2   Basic principles

Applicability

As a research scientist, your purpose is to invent explanations for natural phenomena, contribute them to the pool of competing explanations, and argue their differential credibility. Note that human beings are a part of the natural world, and phenomena involving them may also be construed as natural; so arguments to support or question explanations of human culture or behavior can also be scientific. A scientific approach to the study of human culture and behavior is called social science. The concepts and methods presented here are also applicable to social science.

Argument style

This book is primarily concerned with the argument style that compares observations of natural phenomena (data) to predictions that follow as a logical consequence of a particular explanation. If the observed data are more or less the same as the predictions then we say the data are consistent with that explanation; if the observed data are different from the predictions then we say the data are not consistent with the explanation. Sometimes we describe results more starkly: we say the data fail to disprove an explanation, or we say the data disprove the explanation. Sound scientific argument style evaluates the credibility of any explanation that can make predictions about something observable.

Another argument style, which we might call advocacy, has been common in our western culture for centuries. When practicing advocacy, advocates look for evidence that supports their claim and ignore the rest. Advocates then use only this evidence to formulate arguments that support their claim. Perhaps another person or group does the same for a competing or contradictory claim. Each side presents its evidence and arguments in an effort to convince a third individual or group, or the other side, or even sometimes themselves. Imagine a prosecuting attorney, a defending attorney, and a jury. If both sides were honest and highly skilled, and if the jury were intelligent, attentive, and well informed, then advocacy might contribute to improved understanding. With human nature, however, the desire to win the argument can overwhelm the desire for better understanding. The desire to be on the winning side, or on the side favored by current belief, may be so strong that unpopular or little-known ideas go undefended or even unstated, and thus not fairly tested. Advocacy is not considered an appropriate argument style for science. However, scientific arguments are made by people, and when people care about whether others believe their claims, they tend to include advocacy in their argument style.

When you gather data, you usually have in mind some natural phenomenon you would like to try to explain. You measure instances or cases of the phenomenon and structure them into classes or otherwise recognize relationships among them. The way you make the measurements, construe relationships among the cases, and choose which cases to measure, all help to enable and constrain your explanations. The measurements and their structure constitute a "data set", which can be re-interpreted in the substantive terms of the natural phenomena you are studying.

Structure and variation

Another basic principle discussed in this book is the art of structuring your observations to enable or constrain the formulation and testing of explanations. This will help you create structure and choose observations that will enable you to formulate explanations whose credibility you can asses.

Natural phenomena typically exhibit some variation. When your observations show that things differ, you can wonder why, and invent explanations, called hypotheses, whose differential credibility can then be argued. I recognize three causes of variation: (1) causes that are part of a proposed explanation; (2) causes that are natural, but not described as part of the proposed explanation; and (3) measurement error, caused by the inability to observe or measure accurately. When an explanation simplistically predicts a single value, rarely is the observed value exactly the same as the predicted one, as a consequence of these kinds of variation. To argue against the credibility of an explanation, a predicted value must be sufficiently different from an observed value. A statistical argument quantifies that difference using probability theory. Because of variation, what a hypothesis predicts may not be absolutely clear. What does a hypothesis predict? A statistic describes quantitatively something relevant about the observed data. A statistical hypothesis predicts a probability distribution for a statistic.

The concepts and methods described in this book show how to choose or create statistics and hypotheses that can predict probability distributions for them. This indicates quantitatively the extent to which some aspect of the data is consistent with the hypothesis. Because variation is a part of natural phenomena, as manifest in your measurements and observations, you can legitimately include probability mechanisms as part of your proposed explanations. A statistic is something that you observe or calculate from your data. Choose or invent a statistic that is relevant to the hypothesis you intend to test. Scientific explanations that include hypothesized probability mechanisms can make a prediction that takes the form of a probability distribution for a statistic. Such probability distributions show the probability of the statistic, if your data were generated by the process you hypothesized. By comparing the observed value of the statistic to the probability distribution predicted for it by your hypothesized explanation, you can tell if it is improbably too high or too low, which would argue against the adequacy of your hypothesized explanation.

The methods described in this book show you how to include, as part of your hypothesis, probability mechanisms that you have chosen to represent the variation in the natural phenomenon you would try to explain, and that can work in the context of your data structure. A computer program can instruct a computer to sample your hypothesized probability mechanisms to produce data similar in structure to those you have observed, or intend to observe. These simulated data have values that sample the magnitudes and variability that you have hypothesized. The same statistic that was calculated from your observed data can be calculated in the same way from the simulated data. The frequencies of the thousands of values for a statistic, calculated or observed from thousands of simulated data sets, are arrayed over a horizontal axis labeled with the range of simulated values; this displays the statistic's probability distribution predicted by your hypothesis. This predicted probability distribution gives you a good idea of the range of variation for values of the statistic when your hypothesized mechanism generates data. If the value of the statistic calculated from observed data falls near the middle of this distribution, then the aspect of the data quantified by the statistic is consistent with the hypothesis; if it is off to the side or completely outside this distribution, then it is not consistent with the hypothesis. It is appropriate to interpret this probabilistic comparison, into the more substantive terms of the explanation of the phenomenon in question.

Example of a probability distribution

To make the idea of a probability distribution predicted by a hypothesis a little more concrete, consider this example. I have records of the age at death of hundreds of people who lived (and died) in an urban area of Portugal during the last two decades of the nineteenth century. Of males who lived to be at least three years old, half of them lived to be at least 56 years old. I hypothesize that a late nineteenth-century urban Portuguese male who survives early childhood lives to be at least age 56 with probability 0.5. From a rural agricultural village in the mountainous interior of Portugal, I have age at death records for 14 males who survived early childhood and died during the last two decades of the nineteenth century. I would like to know if these males tend to survive to age 56 better than their urban counterparts. I hypothesize "no", the probability that they will survive to age 56 is 0.5, just like urban males. My test statistic is the number of rural males who survived early childhood and died at age 56 or older. There are 15 possible values (0, 1, .. 14) for this test statistic. For each of these possible values, my hypothesis predicts a probability. You will see the details of how it does this later in this book. Since I have to observe one of these 15 values, the sum of these probabilities is 1.0. These 15 probabilities comprise a probability distribution for the possible values of the test statistic. When I compare the observed number of rural males that survived to age 56 to this predicted probability distribution, it will tell me the probability that I would observe at least that many, or at most that few, if my hypothesis were correct. We call this probability the realized significance of the observed value of the test statistic.

Other argument styles

In addition to this direct comparison of predictions with observations, there are other argument styles that are considered legitimate for science, but these will not be discussed in much depth in this book. One such style, called maximum likelihood, attempts to quantify the exact probability of having observed the data given that a proposed explanation were true; among competing explanations, the one that makes the data seem most likely is favored. Another style, called Bayesian, attempts to quantify the change, when new data are observed, in the prior probabilities that competing hypotheses are true. Once you have mastered the basic probability concepts and hypothesis testing techniques presented in this book, you will be able to study these other argument styles more easily.

1.3   Scientific argument

Ingredients of statistical argument

A scientific argument is directed at increasing or decreasing the credibility of a single explanation of a natural phenomenon, or at increasing the differential credibility of competing explanations of that natural phenomenon. To make a statistical scientific argument, you must formulate a hypothesis that incorporates natural variation in such a way that it predicts a probability distribution for a test statistic whose value you compute from observed data. For this statistical argument to be compelling, you need four basic ingredients: (1) an intellectual foundation that enables you to recognize something to explain and something with which to explain it; (2) structure imposed on the things observed, or on the observations themselves, that enables a clear statement of your hypothesized explanation; (3) a probability mechanism that operates with that structure to generate data similar in form to those you have observed (or will observe), and according to the probability mechanism that you hypothesize to govern how things vary; and (4) a test statistic that can be calculated from the data. In a strict sense, (2) and (3) are your hypothesis, (1) provides the interpretive analogy, and (4) provides something to predict and compare with observations.

Intellectual foundation

Necessary to any scientific argument is something to explain, i.e., variation in something of interest, and something with which to explain it, i.e., variation in observational context to suggest possible explanatory agents. We read publications and talk to one another to learn what has already been observed or credibly argued about a subject of interest. This helps us to recognize both something to explain and possible explanations for it. Training of early career scientists includes much preparation of this kind. Experienced scientists also value time spent, especially near the beginning of a research project, to learn more about the descriptive nature of the phenomena under study and about contextual things of potential relevance. Our work as scientists relies heavily on publications of earlier workers and on interactions with colleagues. Our own preliminary direct observations can also contribute to the intellectual foundation on which more formal data gathering activities and argument rests.

Some of the facts and ideas comprising this intellectual foundation relate to what you want to explain. Other facts and ideas describe the contexts or situations in which the phenomenon to be explained has been or might be observed. Your consideration of both these areas of your intellectual foundation can help you clarify what you want to explain and how you might explain it. This may motivate you to seek more observations in specific relevant contexts. You may find them in published reports, or you may make the observations yourself. These new observations may modify what you want to explain or how you might explain it. This in turn may motivate you to seek more observations … Such an informal process of "reciprocal illumination" characterizes the initial phase of most research projects.

Structure

Eventually, you try to structure these observations, contexts, and ideas into a clear statement of what you want to explain and how you might try to explain it. To some extent, some structure may seem natural to the phenomenon and to your hypothesized explanation of it, but to some extent you invent and impose this structure yourself. Usually there are several ways that the things being observed and the observations themselves can be structured to enable phenomena and hypothesized explanations to be described clearly enough that quantitative predictions can be made. How to create and impose this structure is to some extent an art, because it defies any purely mechanical, operational set of instructions for how to do it. Recognizing, inventing, and imposing structure is part of the larger art form of inventing hypotheses. In consideration of this, the examples in this book are intended to hone your intuition and to give you some tools with which to work creatively, and are not intended to tell you how you have to do it.

Recall the discussion of the kinds of variation that natural phenomena exhibit in relation to an explanation. As you bring your question and possible explanations more clearly into focus, these kinds of variation will distinguish themselves. Some variation may be evident in your observations of the natural phenomena, but legitimately not part of what your hypothesis might explain. Thus, the structure you should impose should serve to ensure that this variation remains constant in data sets construed to be typical of the hypothesis you seek to test. This prevents irrelevant variation from confounding your test. The importance of this will become more clear with the examples in later chapters.

Test statistic

Some of the structure you impose might facilitate the calculation of something that captures an essence of the question you are asking. This something is called a test statistic. If your hypothesis includes a random process to describe some of the variability it seeks to explain, then it predicts a probability distribution of possible values for the test statistic. This predicted probability distribution enables you to discover the probability that the value of the test statistic calculated from your data would be in any given range if the hypothesis were true. This is the basis for hypothesis-testing, statistical arguments in science; if the value of the test statistic calculated from data falls in the middle of the probability distribution predicted for it by your hypothesis, then you argue that (the aspects of) your data (described by the test statistic) are consistent with your hypothesis.

It is important to maintain the conceptual difference between a hypothesis and a test statistic. All by itself, a test statistic is usually just a number that you calculate from data, or trivially calculate by just observing it from data. Usually, the definition of a test statistic does not involve or depend on any hypothesis, except as constrained by the techniques of classical statistics. You may want to define and calculate several different test statistics from the same data. It is possible for a hypothesis to predict for one test statistic a probability distribution with which the observed data are consistent, but predict for another test statistic a probability distribution with which the same observed data are not consistent. Such two test statistics would describe different aspects or facets of the data. Their simultaneous use helps makes more explicit what about the data does or does not seem to be consistent with a proposed explanation. To continue the example of 1.2, I hypothesize that the probability that an urban male who survives early childhood lives to any given age is given by the fraction in my large urban data set of those who do. These probabilities constitute the urban age-at-death distribution. I further hypothesize that the 14 records of age at death for rural males surviving early childhood can be construed as samples of the urban age-at-death distribution. This is a way of hypothesizing that rural age at death is not different from urban age at death. In addition to the test statistic, number of males surviving to age 56, I want to also test the idea that rural folks may be more likely to live to be quite old, so I also use as a test statistic, the number surviving to age 70. You can imagine that the number of rural males surviving to age 56 might fall in the middle of the distribution predicted for it, but if more urban males tended to die in their 60s, then the number of rural males surviving to age 70 would be in the high tail of the distribution predicted for it by the same hypothesis.

You might want to test two different hypotheses to explain the same data. Each hypothesis could predict a different probability distribution for the same test statistic. Somewhere in each of these predicted probability distributions, falls the value of the test statistic calculated from the observed data. Where it falls informs an argument about the differential credibility of the competing explanations. Continuing the same example, my colleague has an age-at-death distribution based on many males who survived early childhood and died near the turn of the twentieth century in rural Spain, over the border from the Portuguese village where I have age-at-death records. Is age at death in rural Portugal more like age at death in rural Spain or in urban Portugal? Each of the two age-at-death distributions can serve as the basis for a hypothesis that predicts its own probability distribution for a test statistic, such as, number of males surviving to age 70, which can be compared to the value observed for it in the rural Portuguese village.

What is a statistical hypothesis?

The structure you impose on the data also enables you to invent or choose a probabilistic data-generating mechanism. When put into action by a computer program, this mechanism generates data with the same structure that you imposed on the observed data. These generated data constitute an example of what you might observe if your hypothesis were true. In a stark, strict sense, taken together, your imposed data structure and your probabilistic data-generating mechanism ARE your hypothesis. In this stark, bare-bones form, the relevance of your hypothesis to the substantive explanation of the real-world phenomena that you seek to explain is achieved by analogy. The structure you impose on the data means things in the real world because you intend for it to mean those things, based on your intellectual foundation.

Your hypothesized probabilistic data-generating mechanism makes clear what things can vary and the probabilistic rules that govern their variation. Your invention or choice of the probabilistic data-generating mechanism used to formulate your hypothesis is your responsibility. Like other aspects of scientific hypothesis creation, this invention or choice is also an art. This book will give you examples to help you get ideas and to stimulate your own creativity, and to provide some instruction in probability theory to give you some basic concepts with which to work. Your statistical argument will carry more weight if you can make clear the analogy between your substantive hypothesized explanation and the probabilistic data-generating mechanism you invent or choose to represent it.

Summary

You need four basic ingredients to make a credible statistical argument: (1) an intellectual foundation; (2) structure imposed on your observations and on the things you observed; (3) a probability mechanism that could operate with that structure to generate data similar in form to those you have observed (or will observe), and according to the probability mechanism that you hypothesize to govern how things vary; and (4) a test statistic that can be calculated from the data to represent something of interest.

You need these ingredients whether you are making a statistical argument using classical techniques, or with the computational approach described in this book. However, once you have these ingredients, you can use your computer to generate a prediction in the form of a probability distribution for the test statistic. To do this you write a program that generates simulated data sets, using the structure and the probabilistic data-generating mechanism you have hypothesized, and that calculates a value for the test statistic for each such data set. Using a thousand or more simulated data sets, a probability distribution for the test statistic can be estimated accurately. This probability distribution is what your hypothesis predicts. When you have calculated the value of your test statistic using your observed data, this predicted probability distribution indicates how surprised you are to have observed such a value given that your hypothesis is true. The interpretive analogy established by ingredient (1) enables your argument about the substantive scientific issues.

At several steps in the process described here, the artistry, creativity, imagination, and pragmatic choices of the scientist must come into play. These same steps also allow the incorporation of irrelevancy, inappropriateness, error, and even dishonesty. Only very rarely have I encountered scientific dishonesty; in every case it occurred by selectively deleting or cleaning data, and not by purposefully manipulating method with the intent to produce a desired result. However, I have encountered many cases of irrelevancy, inappropriateness, or error. A better understanding of method will help us detect and avoid all these problems. The argument styles of scientists are often viewed, especially by non-scientists, as mechanical and objective, in contrast to those of the humanities, which are expected to be more rhetorical and subjective. Scientific argument styles do recognize a distinction between testable and untestable explanations, and do rely on the comparison of data with prediction as a basis for credibility. However, the effective practice of scientific method is a disciplined art, made even more effective when it is explicitly recognized as an art. Scientists themselves contribute to the effectiveness of their art by making explicit what, how, and where inventions, creations, and pragmatic choices enter the formulation of their hypotheses and their test statistics, and the interpretation of their analogies. When a scientific argument has been made, we are each obliged to assess for ourselves the credibility of the hypothesized explanation. When we ourselves make that argument, we sometimes find ourselves among those most difficult to convince of its credibility. At the risk of undermining our own self-confidence, this probably makes a contribution to maintaining the high quality of our own work.

Finally, the most basic goal of this book is to help you practice the art of statistical arguments in science more accurately, more confidently, and more realistically, with the freedom and responsibility that computing power makes available to you.

2 | Programming and statistical concepts

2.1　Computer programming

History

In the late nineteenth and early twentieth century, computing devices became more powerful when they were provided with memory in which to store the data used in the computation. This memory could also store the intermediate results of computation for later use. In the middle of the twentieth century, a major breakthrough in the design of computers occurred when scientists realized that the memory of a computing device could also store the computational instructions themselves. This enabled programmers to compose computational instructions that could be executed automatically, without human intervention.

The instructions that a computer can execute directly need to be very detailed; they are tedious and time consuming to compose, difficult to read even for experienced programmers, prone to errors, and hard to correct. In the late 1950s, some people in the IBM Corporation realized that they could write a computer program that could read statements in a language in which a computer programmer could express his or her intent more efficiently, and then translate those statements into the detailed instructions that a computer can execute directly. We call such a translating program a compiler. Before a compiler can be written, the programming language that it translates, i.e., vocabulary, syntax, and grammar, must be explicitly specified. The program that a compiler translates is called the source statements or source code. When a compiler executes to translate source statements it is said to compile the source statements. The result of a compilation is the object code. Object code is another computer program written with the instructions that the computer can execute directly. When a programmer writes a program in a source language, first source statements are composed using an editor, next those source statements are compiled into object code, and finally that object code is executed to carry out the intent of the programmer. We often use the simpler term, run, to mean execute.

One of the first compilers to be created is called FORTRAN (FORmula TRANslator), and the programming language that it translates is also called FORTRAN. Soon many different compilers had been created, providing programmers with a variety of different programming languages, each intended to meet specific purposes more effectively. One language was designed specifically to teach people programming concepts and good programming techniques. Its structure is fairly simple and its statements are easy to write, read, and correct. This language is called PASCAL; it is the language I used, through the 1990s, to teach the course that produced this book. For reasons I have explained, I now teach this course using spreadsheets, and in this book programming concepts and examples will use spreadsheets.

The instructions that a computer can execute directly usually differ among computers with different central processing units. Compilers for the same source language are often written for different computers, but when computers are too different it is necessary to write in different versions of the same language, or even different languages. With the advent of the internet, programs could be sent easily from one computer to another, but if the computers were too different, the programs would not run on the computer that received them. In the 1990s, Sun Computers developed a programming language called JAVA. JAVA compilers do not compile object code in the native language of any particular computer, but instead compile it into a universal code that can be readily interpreted by a JAVA virtual machine. A JAVA virtual machine is a computer program that interprets and executes JAVA universal code for a particular computer. JAVA virtual machines have been written for nearly every common computer and can be downloaded for free from a Sun Computers web site. This is convenient for computer programmers, because a program written once in JAVA can run on different computers without change. However, the versions of the programming language (BASIC) that EXCEL spreadsheets use for their macros is so similar among different EXCEL versions that macro program text can be cut from one and pasted into another, where it will run with very little (or no) modification. Many other spreadsheet programs, like OpenOffice Calc, use BASIC-like languages for macro programming, although changes are usually necessary for EXCEL macros to run with them.

It is not the purpose of this book to teach you programming beyond the little that you will need to take a computational approach to statistical argument. In the exposition and examples of this book, I will use EXCEL spreadsheets and EXCEL macros, which are computer programs written in EXCEL BASIC. Spreadsheets make it easy to organize data and to present the results of the computation carried out by your macros. Most of you are already familiar with spreadsheets, so mostly you just need to learn how to write macros to carry out calculations.

The two parts of a computer program

A computer program, such as an EXCEL macro, consists of two parts: the first part structures the computer's memory to store data and intermediate results; and the second part provides computational instructions that manipulate data in the computer's memory. All instructions are stored in the computer's memory and executed automatically from there. You compose a program by writing source statements in a programming language. When you run the program, the source statements are translated by a compiler into object code, which is then executed by the computer to carry out your intent.

In EXCEL, where your program is called a macro, you write source statements in the BASIC language, using an editor provided by EXCEL for that purpose. Your source statements are saved when you save a spreadsheet workbook. When you run a macro, its source statements are interpreted, i.e., compiled, but then the object code is run immediately instead of being saved and run later.

Places

A computer program first structures the computer's memory into places. You give each place a name; you will use it to refer to that place in program statements that you will write later. Each place has content (what is stored in that place). Each place has a type that enables the computer to manipulate its content appropriately. The place types that are discussed in this book are named "Integer", "Byte", and "Single". The content of a place of type "Integer" is interpreted as a whole number (positive, negative, or zero). The content of a place of type "Byte" is interpreted as a positive number between 0 and 255 (inclusive), and the content of a place of type "Single" is interpreted as a number with a decimal point, even if it is a whole number. There are many other types of places, but we do not need to know about them to get started with a computational approach to hypothesis formulation and prediction.

You make up names for the places you want to use, and specify the type of each place. You can use any string of characters that begins with a letter and contains no blanks, except for the few words and punctuation characters that are reserved to have pre-defined meaning in the programming language; the names of place types are examples of reserved words. For names of places in the computer's memory, the difference between upper and lower case characters is recognized, i.e., fruit, FRUIT, and FrUiT would all refer to different places. Reserved words are always spelled with an initial uppercase character and subsequent lowercase characters, as with "Integer", "Byte", and "Single", which you have just seen. To help you clearly identify the names of places in the computer's memory, the examples in this book will use all uppercase characters to spell them; all words with any lower case characters are reserved words.

Service berry example

I will illustrate this using a real example that will begin here and conclude in Section 2.3. This example considers the development of ovules into seeds in fruits of the service berry tree, *Amelanchier arborea*. A young developing fruit contains 10 ovules, arranged in 5 enclosures, called carpels, each containing 2 ovules, as shown in Figure 2.1. Some, but usually not all, the ovules develop into seeds. This has evolutionary significance for the service berry tree, which attracts the birds that disperse the seeds in its fruits by offering ripe fruits over a period of many days. The proximal mechanism that enables the service berry tree to do this is that fruits with more seeds ripen sooner than fruits with fewer seeds. The question addressed here is what determines whether an ovule will develop into a seed.

There are several possible explanations for the failure of some ovules to develop into seeds. One class of explanations causes both ovules in a given carpel to develop into seeds or both to abort; a second class of explanations allows each of the two ovules in a carpel to develop into a seed or abort independently of the other. To test whether any explanations in the first class are needed to explain observed data, a macro will instruct the computer to simulate the development of ovules into seeds in service berry fruits, using only the second class of explanations.

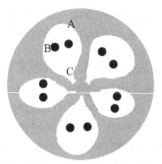

Figure 2.1 Schematic cross section of an *Amelanchier arboria* fruit about 7 mm diameter. A labels one of five carpels; B labels one of two ovules in each carpel; C labels the base of the style for a carpel. Each of the five carpels has its own style leading up to its stigma.

I have given the name FRUIT to a row of 10 places in the computer's memory that will represent a service berry fruit. Each place of FRUIT will represent an ovule; it contains a 1 if the ovule develops into a seed and a 0 if it does not. I will interpret places 1 & 2, 3 & 4, 5 & 6, 7 & 8, and 9 & 10 as representing the five carpels. The values in the 10 places of FRUIT are small non-negative numbers, thus they can be of type "Byte". In programming statements, you can refer to a particular place (ovule) in the row of places called FRUIT in two ways. You can append its sequence number in brackets, e.g., the 3rd place (3rd ovule) in FRUIT would be FRUIT(3), or you can name another place in the computer's memory (I called it OVULE) that holds a sequence number for FRUIT, e.g., if place OVULE contained 3 then the 3rd place in FRUIT would be designated FRUIT(OVULE). Because place OVULE contains a small positive number, it can also be of type "Byte". When writing a macro, you name places and designate their types using the reserved word "Dim", like this:

```
Dim FRUIT(10) As Byte
Dim OVULE As Byte
' FRUIT(OVULE) represents ovule number OVULE of the fruit
' FRUIT(OVULE) contains 1 if that ovule develops into a seed
' FRUIT(OVULE) contains 0 if that ovule aborts
```

"Dim" tells the compiler that you intend to name a place in the computer's memory. After at least one blank, you spell out the name of the place just as you intend to use it later when specifying the computational instructions. If you intend for the name to specify a series of places, such as FRUIT, you append in brackets the number of places in the series. After at least one blank, the reserved word "As" tells the compiler that you intend to specify a type, and after at least one more blank, you specify the type, in these cases "Byte".

The next three lines begin with a single quote; such lines are ignored by the compiler, so you can use them to write messages to yourself about how you intend to interpret places in the computer's memory. It is a good idea to write such messages.

I strongly recommend that in the first part of your macro you name and designate a type for each place you will refer to in the instructions part to follow. This is not actually required by the BASIC interpreter. However, especially if you are not an experienced programmer, it will be useful for you to plan carefully what places in the computer's memory you will need before you start to manipulate their contents, and it will be useful to see, at the beginning of your macro, all the names and types of the places and what you intend for them to mean.

Instructions

After you have named and typed all the places in the computer's memory that you will need, the rest of your program consists of the instructions that manipulate the contents of those places. There are five basic purposes expressed by these instructions:

- change the content of a place in the computer's memory
- perform computation
- change the order in which statements are executed; normally they are executed in the order in which they appear
- read from a spreadsheet or write on a spreadsheet
- cause other sub-programs to execute.

These purposes are often combined in the same statement.

A statement that changes the content of a place in the computer's memory states the name of that place, followed by "=", followed by the new content or by the name of a place containing the new content. For example, the statement

```
OVULE = 3
```

changes the content of the place OVULE; it replaces whatever used to be stored in place OVULE with 3. The statement

```
FRUIT(OVULE) = 1
```

changes the content of the place in FRUIT whose sequence number is the content of OVULE; it replaces it with 1. It is important to realize that there is always something in any place in a computer's memory. Even the number zero is something. If your program has not yet explicitly changed the content of a place that you have named and typed, whatever was in that place when your program began to execute will be in it until its content is changed. Thus it is good practice to give explicitly initial values to all the places that you name. In using statements that change the content of a place in the computer's memory, it is important to be sure that the new content has the appropriate type. For example, do not try to put a decimal point number (type "Single") into OVULE (type "Byte").

Computation often occurs as part of a statement that also changes the content of a place in the computer's memory.

For example, the statement

```
OVULE = OVULE + 1
```

replaces the content of OVULE with the number that is one greater than the number that was already in OVULE. Arithmetic operations are shown with these characters: add "+", subtract "−", multiply "×" and divide "/". Brackets are used as usual to change the order of operations. Although sometimes it is possible to perform arithmetic with the contents of places of different type, e.g., multiply "Single" times "Integer" to get "Single", it is usually safest to perform arithmetic with places of the same type. Some care should be taken to avoid dividing by zero, or generating results that are negative in the case of type "Byte", or too large to fit in the type of space named. In the cases of types "Integer" and "Single", numbers that do not fit are very large indeed.

Normally, statements are executed in the order in which they appear in your program. However, much of the power of computer programs derives from their ability to alter this order, especially to skip or repeat groups of statements. Although there are many kinds of statements that control program flow, i.e., the order in which statements are executed, the examples in this book will use "For .. Next" to repeat a group of statements a given number of times; "Do Until .. Loop" to repeat a group of statements until a specified condition is met; and "If .. Then .. Else" to skip (or not) blocks of statements, depending on whether a specified condition is met.

The use of "For .. Next" takes this form:

```
For OVULE = 1 To 10
    FRUIT(OVULE) = 1
    Next OVULE
```

"For" is followed by the name of a place that has positive "Byte" or "Integer" values, which is followed by "=", followed by the beginning and ending value for that place separated by "To", with everything separated by at least one blank. On subsequent lines are one or more statements. Finally, on its own line is "Next", followed by the same place name that follows "For" on the first line. This causes the one or more statements on the lines between the line with "For" and the line with "Next" to be executed, first with the starting value in OVULE (in this example OVULE contains 1), then with the next value in OVULE (in this example OVULE contains 2), etc. until the statements are executed for a last time with the last value in OVULE (in this example OVULE contains 10). When this so-called "For" loop has finished, all 10 places in FRUIT will contain 1.

The use of "Do Until .. Loop" takes the following form:

```
Do Until (FRUIT(OVULE) = 1)
    OVULE = OVULE + 1
    Loop
```

"Do Until" is followed by an expression that is either true or false. In this example, that statement is

```
FRUIT(OVULE) = 1
```

which is true if in fact the place in FRUIT indicated by the content of place OVULE contains a 1, otherwise it is false. This use of "=" creates a sentence that can be true or false. Another use of "=" means, put a 1 in place FRUIT(OVULE). This creates a sentence that is always true. In an EXCEL macro, you can distinguish these two uses of "=" only by context. Other programming languages, such as PASCAL, do not use "=" to put a value in a place. But now that you are aware that EXCEL's macro programming language has two different meanings for "=", you can try not to be confused. Following the "Do .. Until" on subsequent lines are one or more statements.

Finally on its own line is the reserved word "Loop". The statements in the middle will be executed over and over again until the sentence is true.

In this example, after this so-called "Do Until" loop has executed, OVULE will contain the sequence number of the first place in FRUIT containing 1, i.e., the first ovule in the sequence of ovules in FRUIT to develop into a seed. Of course care must be taken to ensure that at least one place in FRUIT contains a 1, otherwise this Do Until loop would generate an error when the content of OVULE reached 11, because there are only 10 places in FRUIT.

The use of "If .. Then .. Else" statements takes the form:

```
If FRUIT(OVULE) = 0 Then
    (one or more lines of statements)
Else
    (one or more lines of statements)
End If
```

"If" and "Then" bracket a statement that can be true or false. In this example, that statement is

```
FRUIT(OVULE) = 0
```

which gives you another example of the ambiguous use of "=".

On subsequent lines are one or more statements. Next on their own line are the reserved words "End If", or optionally the reserved word "Else". If you choose to use "Else" then it is followed on subsequent lines by one or more statements, finally followed on their own line by the reserved words, "End If". If the statement following the "If" is true, then the statements immediately following, down to the "End If" or the "Else", are executed once. If the statement following the "If" is false, then (if there is an "Else") the statements between "Else" and "End If" are executed once; if there is no "Else", no statements are executed.

Statements that alter flow can be embedded in other statements that alter flow.

In the example below, NOA and NOS are places in the computer's memory of type "Byte". Here, all 10 ovules of the fruit represented by FRUIT are examined; the Number of Ovules that Aborted are counted in place NOA, and the Number of Ovules that became Seeds are counted in place NOS. Before the loop begins, NOA and NOS are initialized by putting 0 in each of them.

```
NOA = 0
NOS = 0
For OVULE = 1 To 10
    If FRUIT(OVULE) = 0 Then
        NOA = NOA + 1
    Else
        NOS = NOS + 1
        End If
    Next OVULE
```

Leading spaces

The macro interpreter ignores leading spaces. This is useful because we can indent groups of statements that will be conditionally skipped or repeated to see more easily which ones they are. Notice how this was done in the preceding examples. Although indentation is not required by the macro interpreter, its practice is highly recommended. As your programs become more complicated, being able to see the structure of the flow will be very useful for correcting mistakes.

Spreadsheet I/O

Your macro programs will read from, and write to, spreadsheets, like this. If R and C are names of places in the computer's memory of type "Integer", then

```
Worksheets("Sheet1").Cells(R,C)
```

refers to the content of the box at row (the content of) R and column (the content of) C of "Sheet1".

Suppose columns 3 through 12 of the 2nd row of "Sheet4" held numbers that were either 0 or 1 to represent the development status of the ovules of a service berry fruit. Those values could be copied to the places of FRUIT in the computer's memory as follows:

```
For C = 3 To 12
    FRUIT(C) = Worksheets("Sheet4").Cells(2,C)
    Next C
```

To write the development status of the ovules of a service berry fruit represented by the places FRUIT in the computer's memory on "Sheet2" in rows 5 through 14 of column 2, we could use the statements

```
For R = 5 To 14
    Worksheets("Sheet2").Cells(R,2) = FRUIT(R)
    Next R
```

Macro statements that read or write are called input/output statements (I/O for short). In other languages, such statements can become quite complicated, especially if they are writing to, or reading from, graphics computer screens, local area networks, web pages, etc. However, our use of a spreadsheet as an I/O interface eliminates the need to learn how to do this sophisticated programming, and enables you to concentrate on the few straightforward programming concepts you can use to do the computation you need to make statistical arguments. Indeed, many experienced programmers use spreadsheet macros and are grateful for the excellent interface that they provide.

Procedures

Variously called Functions, Sub-routines, Methods, etc. in different programming languages, procedures are programs that you (or someone else) have already written. They can be asked to run (called) as part of your program, using names that were given to them by their programmer. You use the name of a procedure as part (or all) of a statement. When your program executes that statement, the procedure named does whatever it is supposed to. There are many procedures (written by other people) already available in the EXCEL macro programming language for you to use in your macros. One that I will use often in this text is called "Rnd". When "Rnd" runs, it produces a uniformly distributed random number of type "Single" between 0.0 and 1.0. If X is the name of a place in the computer's memory of type "Single", the statement

```
X = Rnd
```

puts a random number between 0.0 and 1.0 into place X. The statement

```
X = Rnd * 5.0
```

puts a random number between 0.0 and 5.0 into place X.

You can also write your own procedures (sub-macros), give them a name, and use them in your macros. This is useful because (among other reasons) the name of such a procedure can appear as an instruction in more than one place in your macro, which eliminates the need to copy the same statements into each place. It also lets you see more clearly what your program is intended to do. Other advantages of procedures will become clear when I discuss them in more detail in Section 5.2.

Errors

In composing a program, there are three basic kinds of errors you can make. You can make a mistake in the conventions of the source language, so that the compiler or interpreter becomes confused while trying to compile or interpret your source statements. When this happens, which it does frequently, even with experienced programmers, many programming environments, such as your spreadsheet, return your screen to the editor showing highlighted the source statement where the compiler got confused. As you become more familiar with the syntax of the programming language, you can (usually) easily find and correct the error and run the macro again. The other two basic kinds of errors you can make allow the compiler or interpreter to translate your source statements OK. So-called run-time errors occur while your program is running. An attempt to divide by zero would be an example of a run-time error. The third basic kind of error allows your program to run to completion, but your program does not actually do what you intended. These can be the most dangerous kinds of errors because they can remain undetected, causing your program to provide you with wrong results. Techniques to ensure that your program is doing what you intend, and for finding and correcting errors, will be presented in the examples and exercises to follow.

2.2   You start programming

Experienced programmers

You have read about the basic principles of a computational approach to statistical argument, and some basic concepts in computer programming, and you have been exposed to some of the language conventions that EXCEL provides for you to program macros. Now you will start programming for yourself. This section deals explicitly with how to program EXCEL macros to implement a computational approach to statistical argument. If you are an experienced EXCEL macro programmer, you can skip this section. If you are an experienced programmer of another language, e.g., JAVA, and prefer to program in that language, you can skip this section, and treat the examples to follow as pseudocode. However, many experienced programmers have discovered that for small programs, as those in this text will be, EXCEL macros can be very convenient, so you may want to read this section anyway.

Getting started with EXCEL macro programming

EXCEL 2008 for MAC does not allow macro programming, so if you are a MAC user, you need to have an earlier version of EXCEL, or work on a WINDOWS machine. EXCEL 2007 for WINDOWS appears not to allow macro programming, but in fact it does. If you have EXCEL 2007 for WINDOWS, open EXCEL and click the office button in the upper left corner. In the bottom right of the window that opens, click "Excel Options". Near the top of the window that opens, click to check "Show Developer tab in the Ribbon" and then click "OK". At the top center of the EXCEL spreadsheet click the developer tab, which should now be showing. At the far left click "Visual Basic". You should now be in the macro development environment.

If you have EXCEL for WINDOWS 2004 or earlier, open EXCEL, bring down the "Tools" menu, and click on "Macros", which opens the "Macros" menu. Three choices in this menu are relevant to our purpose: "Macros", "Security" and "Visual Basic Editor". Click on "Macros" to open a window that lists current macros; at present, you should see an empty list. Click on "Security" to open a window with two tabs: "Security level" and "Trusted sources". Select "Medium" security. You should be the only one writing macros for the workbooks that you will save, so leave the list of trusted sources blank, and check the "Trust all" box at the bottom. This could be the last time you will have to visit "Security". You might want to visit the "Macros" list to re-run a macro that you have already written. Mostly, you will open and use the Visual Basic Editor (VBE). Versions of EXCEL for MAC and some versions of EXCEL for WINDOWS may differ slightly from the description I have presented here of how to access VBE, but if you experiment a little you will discover how to open VBE on your computer.

In this text, I will present only a small sub-set of the power and language of Visual Basic, so you do not need to learn much about Visual Basic to learn how to write macros to implement computational approaches to statistical argument using EXCEL. You will find in this text all you need to know. Most students who have gotten a Visual Basic book and tried to learn Visual Basic while trying to study this text have found it counterproductive.

When you are ready to try, open your VBE. The screen should show a column on the left, divided into an upper window called "VBA Project" and a lower window called "Properties"; there also may be a short, wide window across the rest of the bottom of the screen called "Watches", above which may be shown a large blank space, which becomes the editor when you create or choose something to edit. You can open or close these windows yourself, so the windows showing at any given time can vary. In VBE, bring down the "Insert" menu and click on "Module". Another branch, terminating in the word, "Module1", will be added to the tree of objects and to the modules in the "Project" window in the upper left. If the word, "Module1", is not already highlighted in this tree, click on it to highlight it. The large blank space to the right will light up; this space has now become your macro editor. In the window in the lower left, the word, "Module1", appears on the first line after the word, "Name". Click on this line in the blank space to enable a write cursor. Use your keyboard to erase the word, "Module1", and write the word, TRY. Click again in the "Project" window above; the word, "Module1", in the tree becomes the word TRY. Click in the macro editor (the large space to the upper right) to enable the write cursor.

Use your keyboard to type the characters

```
Sub TRY()
```

if they are not already there. When you press the Enter key, the characters, "End Sub", (usually) automatically appear below the write cursor. At the write cursor, type the characters,

```
MsgBox ("Begin TRY")
```

As you do so, a small box may open to remind you of the syntax associated with this statement, which will go away when you press the Enter key. You may find these reminders useful later, but for now just ignore them. Now type on the next line the characters

```
MsgBox ("End TRY")
```

Pay attention to type the upper and lower cases and the blanks exactly as shown. If things are not just right, EXCEL will not understand; when you try to run the macro, characters in the editor will turn red where EXCEL could not understand you. Often this will be near where you have made a mistake, so you can look for your mistake nearby, find it and correct it. Click the mouse below the last line with the characters, "End TRY". Now bring down the "Run" menu and click "Run Sub". If your macro runs, you have just written and run a macro. When this macro runs, a spreadsheet is shown with a message box that says, "Begin TRY" with an "OK" button below it. Click the "OK" button. Now another message box is shown that says "End TRY" with an "OK" button below it. Click the "OK" button. You should now be back in the VBE macro editor.

This is a good time to bring down the file menu and click on "Save Book1. xls", which is actually a "Save as" that will let you browse to a location. Choose the desktop and save "Book1.xls" as "TRY.xls". Close EXCEL and look on the desktop for the icon for "TRY.xls". Click it open. EXCEL will open with it. Pull down the "Tools" menu; click on "Macros"; in the "Macros" menu click on "Macros" to see the list of your macros. Now macro, TRY, should be on your list. Click on the "Run" button in the upper right to run the macro again. If you have not yet seen any red in the macro editor, go now to the macro editor. The program statements for macro, TRY, should already be showing in the editor, but if not click on "Module", TRY, in the tree in the Project window in the upper left. Erase the first quote mark from the statement

```
MsgBox ("Begin TRY")
```

and then click below the last line to see red (probably) in your editor, together with a message suggesting what might be wrong. Sometimes these suggestions are helpful, but often they do not tell you very clearly what you need to fix, so do not take them too literally. What they do tell you for sure is that something is wrong and you have to fix it. Sometimes EXCEL does not know that it is going to get confused by one of your errors until it tries to run your macro. In this case the macro stops running where EXCEL got confused and returns you to the macro editor with red near where EXCEL got confused, which may be near what you have to fix, but if not then your error will almost always have been made before the red characters. The gentle art of fixing programs is an important dimension of a programmer's skill, and develops with experience. So be patient and expect to make mistakes; after decades of experience, I still make many.

How to read and write a spreadsheet from your macro

One thing that is convenient about using EXCEL macros for a computational approach to statistical argument is that your macro can read and write directly from a spreadsheet, as you have seen from the examples of statements in the preceding section. So you can do that yourself now. Open TRY.xls, ensure that you have "Sheet1" showing, and enter your age in years into the cell in the first row and second column. Save the spreadsheet and open VBE. Your statements for macro, TRY, should appear in the macro editor, but if they do not then click on TRY, in the "Project" window. Press the Enter key after the line

```
MsgBox ("Begin TRY")
```

to open a blank space below, and type into it these lines:

```
'Name and type a place in the computer's memory to hold my age
   Dim MYAGE As Integer
'Read my age into that place from cell Row 1, Col 2 of Sheet1
   MYAGE = Worksheets("Sheet1").Cells(1,2)
'Write the contents of MYAGE into cell Row 2, Col 3 of Sheet2
   Worksheets("Sheet2").Cells(2,3) = MYAGE
```

Click after the last line (it should contain "End Sub"). Now bring down the "Run" menu and run your macro. After you have clicked the "OK" button in the "End TRY" message box, go back to the spreadsheets and open "Sheet2" to see your age in the cell at row 2, col 3.

In your macro editor, any characters following a single prime up to the end of the line are comments; they are ignored by EXCEL when you run your macro, but they remind you of what you intend for the statements in your macro to mean or do. Open your macro editor, if it is not open already, and notice that comments are shown in a different color, often green, so you can distinguish them more easily from program statements. You should associate with nearly every executable statement a comment that explicitly says what you intend for it to mean or do. Being aware of your intent will help you find and correct your mistakes, which will be much more difficult to do without such comments. While you are composing your program and have your intent more fully in mind, comments, indentation, use of upper and lower case letters, and other stylistic considerations may seem redundant. You may feel annoyed by this redundancy, but please be patient. Many of my students, including some of the most brilliant, have come to appreciate this redundancy, especially as their efforts to grasp concepts begin to produce more confidence. When you have mastered the sections of Chapter 2, you will have nearly all you need (except practice) to write confidently EXCEL macros to take a computational approach to statistical argument.

2.3 Completing the service berry example

Fruit-ripening phenology

In the late 1980s at the University of Michigan, David Gorchov's Ph.D. thesis research sought to explain variation in the length of the period during which some woody plants that produce berry-like fruits present them to potential dispersers. Some plants, like *Prunus virginiana* (choke cherry) present their ripe fruits all within a few days. This tends to attract generalist dispersers, who come in large numbers during these few days to take advantage of the copious supply of food. Other plants, such as the woody vine, *Solanum dulcamara* (night shade), present a few ripe fruits in early summer and continue to do so until the growing tips of their branches are killed by frost in the fall. This schedule of fruit presentation trains a few specialist dispersers to visit the plant many different days on a regular basis to exploit a small but reliable food source. *Amelanchier arborea* (a service berry relative) is a small understory tree with bird-dispersed, berry-like fruits, which ripen on different days during a few weeks in late spring and early summer, to attract somewhat more reliable and specialized dispersers.

Scientists seek evolutionary (ultimate) explanations for why a plant would benefit from a longer or shorter period of time during which it presented fruits to potential dispersers. These benefits might have to do with attracting specialist or generalist dispersers, or with the reliability of a disperser's presence at specific times of year, or with avoiding disease or thieves at other times of year. Scientists also seek mechanistic (proximal) explanations for how a plant might control when its fruits ripen, whatever might be the benefits for this timing.

Mechanisms of variation in fruit-ripening date

David's research dealt with both kinds of explanations and a number of different study organisms. The example that we will examine in more detail here concerns his evaluation of mechanistic explanations for how *Amelanchier arborea* creates variation in ripening date among its fruits. He gathered data to show that the number of ovules that develop into seeds as fruits mature is highly variable among fruits of the same tree. He showed that development time from pollination to maturity for a fruit is closely correlated with the number of seeds in the fruit: those fruits with more seeds develop more rapidly, as if in consequence of a stronger resource "sink" messaged by the greater hormone production of more plant embryos. Seed number remained variable among the fruits on a tree, even under experimental conditions when flowers were provided with excess pollen or stems bearing developing fruits were defoliated or partially girdled. It seems plausible that *Amelanchier arborea* may be maintaining its variation in fruit-ripening date on purpose, as it were, by maintaining variation in seeds per fruit. Thus, David directed his attention to testing hypotheses suggesting various mechanisms that might result in varying numbers of seeds among the fruits of *Amelanchier arborea*.

The various hypotheses to explain the mechanisms by which the plant might maintain variation in the number of seeds that mature in any given fruit can be divided into two broad types, best understood by considering the anatomy of the developing fruits of *Amelanchier arborea*. Each fruit has five carpels and each carpel has two ovules and one style, as has been shown in Figure 2.1. Potentially, every ovule could develop into a seed, to produce

10 seeds in a fruit. Some mechanisms might cause each carpel to be affected individually by things that would interfere equally with the development of both of its ovules. For example, a non-functional style would result in no pollination and cause both ovules to abort (not become seeds). Such mechanisms that operate at the level of the whole carpel David called carpel-mediated mechanisms. Other mechanisms might vary in intensity from fruit to fruit, but affect the ovules within a fruit without regard to their carpel membership. For example, the level of nutrients available to the whole fruit might vary, with those near leaves in sunnier positions receiving more than those near leaves in shadier positions. The chance that an ovule develops into a seed might be greater in a fruit in a sunnier place, but that chance would be the same for all ovules in the same fruit, and they would realize that chance independently of other ovules in the same or a different carpel. Such mechanisms that operate at the level of the whole fruit are called fruit-mediated mechanisms.

David hypothesized a number of mechanisms, and in this way identified each as carpel mediated or fruit mediated. In carpel-mediated mechanisms, both ovules in a carpel were hypothesized to develop into seeds or abort with a probability that could differ among carpels. In fruit-mediated mechanisms, the chances that an ovule developed into a seed differed among fruits, but within a fruit it was hypothesized to be the same for all ovules without regard to the success of their carpel mate or the other ovules.

The data

To gather data to test the differential credibility of these two kinds of hypotheses, David collected hundreds of fruits at a variety of developmental stages, embedded them in paraffin by passing them through an alcohol dehydration series, cut them into thin sections with a microtome, and looked at them under a light microscope. Unfortunately, the carpel walls disintegrate as the fruit matures, so that when the seeds are fully mature, the carpel walls can no longer be seen in a microscopic section. The carpel walls are clearly visible early in the maturation of the fruit, but at that time it is not yet clear which ovules are destined to actually develop into seeds. There is a very small window of opportunity in the development of fruits when both seeds and carpel walls can be seen together in a microscopic section. Such fruits must be collected at just the right stage.

Most fruits were not quite at the right stage, but after much effort David observed seeds in the ovules of 43 fruits. It takes weeks to prepare fruits and section them. By the time fruits could be observed, the fruiting season was over, and the option of collecting and preparing even more fruits was no longer available. The large amount of unproductive work involved makes collecting more fruits an unattractive option in any case. Such considerations of limited field season and observational difficulties are typical of organismal studies. Most original research in natural science has similar challenges that limit the amount and quality of data. A strong desire to be able to reason as powerfully as possible with the limited data available motivates the use of a computational approach to statistical argument.

Location of seeds in 43 fruits of *Amelanchier arborea*									
Number of seeds	3	4	5	6	7	8	9	10	
Total no. fruits with that many seeds	14	5	4	3	3	3	4	7	43
Number of seeds in those fruits	42	20	20	18	21	24	36	70	251
No. of carpels with two seeds	7	4	5	5	9	10	16	35	91
No. of carpels with one seed	28	12	10	8	3	4	4	0	69

It is useful to make some observations about this data structure. There are no fruits with fewer than three seeds. Most fruits that do not have at least three seeds are aborted by the parent plant and drop to the ground before they begin to develop, probably to save the plant the cost of making an expensive fruit to attempt to disperse so few seeds. The first row times the second row equals the third row. The third row equals twice the fourth row plus the fifth row. The 43 fruits contain 430 ovules and 215 carpels, in 91 of which both ovules developed into seeds.

Hypothesis and statistic

The hypothesis that only carpel-mediated mechanisms, in which both seeds in a carpel succeed or fail together, predicts that no carpels with only one seed would ever be observed. But 69 such carpels were observed. So it would seem that carpel-mediated mechanisms cannot explain all the variation. Are carpel-mediated mechanisms needed at all, or could fruit-mediated mechanisms be sufficient? To answer this question David hypothesized that only fruit-mediated mechanisms produced the variation in number of seeds in a fruit.

To make this a statistical hypothesis, he needed to choose (invent, define) a test statistic, and to make explicit a probability mechanism that he could sample to calculate an example data set that would be typical of what he might have observed if the hypothesized mechanism had actually generated his data. A data set calculated in this way is often called a simulated data set. A value of the test statistic is calculated using this example data set. Many such typical data sets are independently calculated, each time also calculating a value for the test statistic. This collection of values constitutes a prediction of the hypothesis about the range of variation of the test statistic. This prediction approximates a probability distribution for the test statistic. If the observed value of the test statistic falls in the middle of the predicted range of variation, then the aspect of the data described by the test statistic is consistent with the hypothesis. In our example, the hypothesis is that variation in numbers of seeds can be explained by fruit-mediated mechanisms. If the observed value of the test statistic falls near one of the extremes (or entirely outside) of the predicted range of variation, then it would seem unlikely that the hypothesized mechanism could have generated the observed data; other explanations might be more appropriate.

David wanted to choose a test statistic that was relevant to the question under consideration, are fruit-mediated mechanisms adequate to explain the observed data? David chose the total number of carpels with two seeds as his test statistic. From his data structure, he observed its value, 91. This test statistic is a good choice because if the number of carpels with two seeds were too high or too low to be consistent with numbers predicted by fruit-mediated mechanisms, it would enable the argument that carpel-mediated mechanisms may also affect the number of seeds in a fruit.

David needed to explicitly define a probability mechanism that can generate data that have the same structure, and that credibly represent the idea of fruit-mediated mechanisms. He wanted the simulated data sets to look just like his data structure, except for variation that is directly relevant to the hypothesized explanation in question. The question is not about how many fruits have been observed, so the hypothesized probability mechanism should generate data structures with 43 fruits. The question is not even about how many fruits were observed with a given number of seeds, so the hypothesized probability mechanism should generate data structures in which the number of fruits with a given number of seeds is exactly the same as the number of fruits observed with that number of seeds. Any probability mechanism that did not do this would result in a less convincing statistical argument. Fruit-mediated probability mechanisms are those by which the number of seeds that did develop in a fruit, developed from any of the ovules with equal probability. David chose a fruit-mediated probability mechanism that generates a three-seeded fruit by choosing equiprobably any 3 of the 10 ovules to become seeds; a four-seeded fruit by choosing equiprobably any 4 of the 10 ovules to become seeds etc. To generate a data set, 14 three-seeded fruits, 5 four-seeded fruits, etc. up to seven 10-seeded fruits would be generated in this way. For each such data structure, the test statistic is calculated, i.e., count the number of two-seeded carpels.

A macro to calculate the predicted probability distribution

To write a macro to calculate a data set typical of David's hypothesized fruit-mediated mechanisms, I needed to reserve places in the computer's memory that represent an *Amelanchier arborea* fruit with 10 ovules. In the example macro here, I invented the name, FRUIT, for the place that represents a fruit, and said how many units of data it can hold (10), and how to interpret each of those data units, As Byte, like this:

```
Dim FRUIT(10) As Byte
```

I interpret the places as ovules, and intend for a place to contain 1 if that ovule develops into a seed, and 0 if it aborts. Notice that the meaning of the contents of the 10 places of FRUIT depends entirely on what I intend for them to mean. Thus, if FRUIT(3) contains 1, it means to me that the third ovule, which is the first ovule in the second carpel, developed into a seed.

   To manipulate a data structure typical of a hypothesized fruit-mediated mechanism, it is useful to be able to refer to particular ovules indirectly, using another place in the computer's memory to serve as an index for FRUIT. I have called this place OVULE. I named and typed it like this:

```
Dim OVULE As Byte
```

For example, if OVULE contains 3, then FRUIT(OVULE) is intended to contain the development status of the third ovule.

Before my macro can use the places, FRUIT() and OVULE, to refer to the information in a data set typical of the fruit-mediated hypothesized mechanisms, I must program my macro to put information in them. All the computer needs to know to generate a data set is how many fruits there are with a given number of seeds. I have entered this information in the first 10 rows of the first column of "Sheet1" of a spreadsheet; my macro will instruct the computer to read from there. I named a place R As Byte to index the rows of the spreadsheet, and a place NFL As Byte to represent the Number of Fruits Left (with R seeds) to generate in a simulated data set. Each time my macro simulates a fruit it will count the Number of carpels with a Pair of seeds and accumulate the total number in a place that I have named NP As Byte. When an entire data set has been simulated, NP will hold the value of the test statistic for that data set. Next, I composed statements that would simulate a data set, leaving the details of how to compute a random fruit with R seeds, and of how to count the number of carpels with a pair of seeds in that data set, as yet unspecified. By composing these details later, I can now see the flow of my macro more easily to ensure that it does what I intend. When I do compose these details, I will put them in their places.

My instructions so far look like this:

```
NP = 0
For R = 3 To 8
   NFL = Worksheets("Sheet1").Cells(R,1)
   Do Until NFL = 0
      Statements to generate a random fruit with R seeds
      Statements to count Number of carpels with a Pair of
      seeds and increment NP
   NFL = NFL - 1
   Loop
Next R
NP = NP + Worksheets("Sheet1").Cells(9,1) * 4
NP = NP + Worksheets("Sheet1").Cells(10,1) * 5
```

For each value of R from 3 to 8, my macro reads from "Sheet1" into place NFL the number of fruits with (the content of) R seeds that need to be simulated. Then (in ways not yet specified) it simulates a fruit with (the content of) R seeds, and each carpel in that fruit with a pair of seeds increments (the content of) NP. Then it decrements (the content of) NFL to indicate how many fruits with (the content of) R seeds it still has left to simulate. If it had any left, it simulates another fruit with (the content of) R seeds. When NFL finally contains 0, the computer will know to stop simulating fruits with (the content of) R seeds. These repeated simulations are implemented with a "Do Until . . Loop". Then my macro puts the next higher number into R and reads from "Sheet1" into NFL the number of fruits with (the now one higher content of) R seeds. Then those fruits are simulated and each carpel with a pair of seeds increments (the content of) NP. These calculations are repeated over and over until fruits with eight seeds have been simulated and (the content of) NP appropriately incremented. These repeated calculations are implemented with the "For R = 3 To 8 . . Next R" block of statements, which contains a "Do Until . . Loop" block of statements, with each block respectively indented. My macro does not have to simulate 9- or 10-seeded fruits because 9-seeded fruits always have four 2-seeded carpels and 10-seeded fruits always have five 2-seeded carpels. The last two statements increment (the content of) NP by reading the number of 9- and 10-seeded fruits from "Sheet1" and multiplying by 4 or 5. Now, NP contains the value of the test statistic for a data set with exactly the same numbers of fruits with given numbers of seeds as David's original data set, but simulated under the hypothesis that the seeds that did develop could have developed equiprobably from any of the 10 ovules without regard to their carpel membership.

These statements generate one simulated data set and thus one simulated value for the test statistic, held in NP. I intend for my macro to simulated 1000 such values for the number of carpels with a pair of seeds (the test statistic) and write them onto "Sheet1" to estimate the probability distribution for the test statistic predicted by the hypothesis that seeds develop equiprobably without regard to carpel membership. To do this I put all the statements above in a "For .. Next" loop that executes 1000 times to calculate 1000 simulated values for the test statistic. Each time a data set is simulated, its value for the test statistic, held in NP, is written in the second column of "Sheet1". When my macro is finished running, I will ask EXCEL to sort the values in the second column of "Sheet1". This will produce an estimated predicted probability distribution for the test statistic. Because 1000 values were simulated, the value in row 500 is at the middle of the distribution; the value in row 100 is at the 10th percentile etc.

To implement my intent, I named a place, NS, of type "Integer" to count the number of simulations. Now the instruction part of my macro looks like this:

```
For NS = 1 To 1000
    All the statements above
    Worksheets("Sheet1").Cells(NS,2) = NP
    Next NS
```

Notice that the first statement in the block "All the statements above" re-initializes NP with 0, and that the place NS not only counts simulations in the "For NS . . Next" block, but also indicates the row of column 2 in "Sheet1" where the next simulated value of the test statistic is written.

To finish my macro, I still need to compose statements to simulate a fruit with (content of) R seeds placed in some (content of) R of its ovules chosen equiprobably at random, and then to identify carpels with a pair of seeds to increment (the content of) NP. The first task starts by putting (the content of) R 1s in the first (the content of) R places of FRUIT and 0s in the rest.

My statements look like this:

```
For OVULE = 1 To R
    FRUIT(OVULE) = 1
    Next OVULE
For OVULE = R+1 To 10
    FRUIT(OVULE) = 0
    Next OVULE
```

By now, you should be able to recognize "For . . Next" blocks, and imagine how they work. Suppose that R contains 5. Take a piece of paper and draw a tall narrow rectangle of 10 squares one above the other to represent FRUIT() in the computer's memory. Label the 10 squares with the numbers 1, 2, . . 10. These labels represent possible values in R. Now you execute these statements, as if you were the computer, writing a 0 or 1 in each of the 10 squares. Did you end up with 1s in the first five squares and 0s in the last five?

Random re-arrangement – Next, my macro will choose a random re-arrangement of all 10 places by randomly swapping the contents of the 10 places. I name a place, NOL, of type "Byte", to represent the Number of Ovules Left to swap, and a place, X, of type "Single", to load with a uniformly distributed random number to choose the next place to swap. A place named HOLD holds the contents of a place to swap so that they are not lost when the new contents are put there. My statements to choose a random re-arrangement look like this:

```
NOL = 10
Do Until NOL = 1
    X = Rnd * NOL
    OVULE = 1
    Do Until OVULE > X
        OVULE = OVULE + 1
    Loop
    If OVULE <> NOL Then
        HOLD = FRUIT(OVULE)
        FRUIT(OVULE) = FRUIT(NOL)
        FRUIT(NOL) = HOLD
    End If
    NOL = NOL - 1
Loop
```

This block of statements permutes the 10 places of FRUIT so that one of the possible $10 \times 9 \times .. \times 2$ re-arrangements is chosen equiprobably. Such a re-arrangement is called a permutation. These statements implement my intent to choose a permutation equiprobably. They work like this. One of the remaining unswapped ovules (initially any of the 10) is chosen equiprobably, using the procedure "Rnd" (provided by VBE): first a random number uniformly distributed between 0.0 and 1.0 is generated by "Rnd" and then multiplied by (the content of) NOL and placed in X. To serve as an index for FRUIT(), this number needs to be converted to type "Byte" and put in Ovule, a place of type "Byte". That place will be place OVULE. My macro initializes OVULE with the value 1; then using a "Do Until .. Loop", keeps incrementing (the content of) OVULE (if necessary) until it exceeds (the content of) X. OVULE now contains an index for FRUIT() chosen equiprobably among the numbers from 1 to (the content of) NOL. My macro will now swap the development status of FRUIT(OVULE) with that of FRUIT(NOL). If (the content of) OVULE is the same as (the content of) NOL, then (obviously) no swap is necessary, else my macro puts (the content of) FRUIT(OVULE) into place HOLD, so that it will not be lost when (the content of) FRUIT(NOL) is put into place FRUIT(OVULE), and finally (the content of) HOLD is put into place FRUIT(NOL). The development status (content) of FRUIT(NOL) is now part of the permutation, because the next instruction decrements (the content of) NOL to consider only the ovules in the first NOL places of FRUIT during the next iteration of the "Do Until . . Loop". When there is only one unswapped ovule left, there is nothing to swap, so FRUIT() now contains an equiprobably chosen permutation of the development status of its ovules. Choosing a permutation equiprobably is a probability mechanism that you will find useful later in formulating your own hypotheses.

Calculate the test statistic

Finally, for each fruit, my macro discovers the number of carpels with a pair of seeds and increments NP accordingly, using a place, B, of type "Byte", to identify carpels, like this:

```
B = 2
For OVULE = 1 To 10
    If B = 2 Then
        B = 1
    Else
        B = 2
    End If
    If B = 2 Then
        NP = NP + FRUIT(OVULE-1) * FRUIT(OVULE)
    End If
    Next OVULE
```

These statements illustrate somewhat more sophisticated programming techniques to perform tasks like this, so be patient with yourself as you try to understand them. You may find it useful to take out your piece of paper again, to execute the statements yourself as if you were the computer. Usually, when I am designing and checking a block of statements to perform a particular task, I take out a piece of paper, mark squares and sequences of squares, and then execute my statements as if I were the computer. You will find that this is a useful technique later when you design your own macros in the context of your own research. In the statements above, the test sentence, "If B = 2", identifies when OVULE contains an even index for FRUIT(). Because I intend for every two ovules in FRUIT to represent a carpel, when (the content of) OVULE is even, I know that (the content of) FRUIT(OVULE-1) and FRUIT(OVULE) represent the development status of two ovules in the same carpel. The product of these contents will be 1 only when both ovules develop into seeds, else it will be 0. In this way I can ask my macro to increment NP by this product to count the number of carpels with a pair of seeds.

Remember the four ingredients

David's example illustrates the four basic ingredients that you will need to formulate a hypothesis that incorporates natural variation in such a way that you can use computation to estimate the probability distribution for your test statistic predicted by your hypothesis, to compare with observed data.

These ingredients are:

(1) Knowledge of the basic biology. The anatomy, development, physiology, ripening phenology, bird dispersal agents, etc. of *Amelanchier arborea* fruits presents constraints and enables David to impose structure to clearly describe how different classes of hypothesized mechanisms might have generated his observed data. Some of the research to understand this biology had been done before David began his own investigation. He had to know about this before he could ask his own questions, even though his own research would make substantial contributions. However, even with the basic biology in place, choices of how to impose structure on the data remain.

(2) Data structure. In David's test of seed maturity hypotheses in *Amelanchier arborea*, he structured his data as 43 fruits, each with 10 ovules in 5 carpels of 2 each; for each ovule, whether or not it developed into a seed was noted. He counted the number of carpels with two seeds and chose to use that as his test statistic. You, the researcher, structure your observations; this does not happen by itself. How you structure your observations can influence substantially what questions you can ask and how you can ask them. In subsequent sections of this text, you will see a variety of data structures that will help develop your ability to structure productively the observations you make in your own research. Ultimately, structuring data is part of the art of the effective practice of science.

(3) Hypothesized probability mechanism. To represent fruit-mediated mechanisms, David hypothesized that for a fruit with R seeds, any way of choosing which R of the 10 ovules would develop into a seed

was equally likely, and he used this mechanism to generate data sets having the same number of fruits with R seeds as observed. This is one of a number of possible probability mechanisms that could have been used to represent hypothesized variation. As part of his scientific argument, David points out that this hypothesized probability mechanism does not introduce irrelevant variation, but does represent the idea of fruit-mediated mechanisms to determine the number of seeds in a fruit.

(4) Test statistic. The number of carpels with two seeds was chosen as the test statistic to test hypotheses about seed maturation mechanisms in *Amelanchier arborea*. This was a good choice because its extreme values indicate dependence of the maturation of the two ovules in the same carpel. The imposition of data structure that recognized carpel membership for mature seeds enabled the calculation (count) of the value of this test statistic. The number of carpels with two seeds is a relevant test statistic, so David can use it to make a relevant argument based on its predicted probability distribution. As you will see in Section 3.1, sometimes scientists mistakenly argue about test statistics that are not very related to the proposed explanations. In the past, the choice of test statistic was often severely constrained by the need to use pre-calculated probability distributions. David's predicted probability distribution for the number of two-seeded carpels did not resemble any of the pre-calculated probability distributions of classical statistics. By explicitly calculating predicted probability distributions, your choice of test statistics need no longer be limited to those described by classical statistics; you can choose test statistics that are easy to observe or calculate, and that have clear meaning in your scientific explanations.

If you are feeling somewhat overwhelmed by this example, please do not despair. I do not expect you to master all its details at the first reading. One purpose of this section is to give you a good look at the approach of this book, which will help you to formulate specific hypotheses, and to use computation to predict from them probability distributions for test statistics that will enable you to quantify their consistency with observed data. You may want to revisit this example after you have had more practice with the concepts. The other purpose of this and the preceding sections, together with the next section, which shows my entire macro, CARPEL, is to be your EXCEL macro computing manual. In these sections, most of the programming language concepts and conventions that you will need for the rest of the book have been presented. I do not expect you to remember everything; I do not remember everything myself. I do expect you to consult these explanations and examples frequently as you read the rest of the text, and as you go on to write your own macros.

Name vs content

You have noticed throughout the preceding sections the repeated use of (the content of) in association with references to names of places in the computer's memory. A very important concept that is often challenging to beginning programmers is the distinction between the name of a place and its contents. This is made even more challenging by the tendency of experienced programmers to use the name of a place to mean either the place or its contents, depending on context. Once you have grasped the distinction and can recognize the context, it is annoying to keep saying (the content of). So in the rest of this text, if X (for example) is the name of a place in the computer's memory, references to X will mean either the place or its content, depending on context. You can refer to your programming manual (this Chapter 2) to be reminded how to tell.

If you would like to learn more about David's study, you are invited to read Gorchov and Estabrook (1987).

2.4   Sub CARPEL

Sub CARPEL()

'Carpel reads from column 1 of "Sheet1" the number of fruits
'with "row" number of ovules that develop seeds.
'For each fruit, randomly assigns its seeds to ovules
'Construes the 5 carpels as ovules 1&2, 3&4 etc.
'Counts the number NP of 2 seeded carpels in the data set.
'Writes NP for simulation NS in row NS column 2 of Sheet1

```
Dim FRUIT(10) As Byte
Dim OVULE As Byte
' FRUIT(OVULE) represents ovule number "contents of OVULE"
' FRUIT(OVULE) has 1 if this ovule becomes a seed else 0

Dim NFL As Byte
'NFL has the number of fruits with "row" seeds left to simulate

Dim X As Single
Dim NOL, HOLD As Byte
'X has a random number
'NOL has the number of ovule positions left to choose among
'HOLD is used to swap values in FRUIT during permutation

Dim R As Byte
' Index to read or write worksheet cell at row R

Dim NP As Byte
'NP is number of 2-seeded carpels
'NP is counted over the whole data set.
'NP is the test statistic

Dim B As Byte
'B identifies each pair of ovules (a carpel) in a fruit

Dim NS As Integer
' NS is the number of simulations completed so far

'instructions to manipulate the contents of these places

MsgBox ("Begin Carpel")

'Whatever follows MsgBox in quotes between parens
'is written in a message box on the spreadsheet

Randomize
'Simulate 1000 data sets
```

```
For NS = 1 To 1000
'Initialize random number generator

'Initialize number of 2-seeded carpels to count all the
'fruits in this simulated data set.
'NP will contain the test statistic
   NP = 0

'For each of the possible number R of seeds in a fruit
   For R = 3 To 8

'Read the number of fruits with R seeds from Sheet1 column 1
      NFL = Worksheets("Sheet1").Cells(R,1)
      Do Until NFL = 0
'Until there are no fruits left, generate a fruit with R seeds
         For OVULE = 1 To R
            FRUIT(OVULE) = 1
            Next OVULE
         For OVULE = R + 1 To 10
            FRUIT(OVULE) = 0
            Next OVULE

'Permute the contents of the ovule positions in FRUIT
         NOL = 10
'NOL is the number of ovule positions left to choose among
         Do Until NOL = 1
            X = Rnd * NOL
'Randomly select one of the first NOL places in FRUIT
            OVULE = 1
            Do Until OVULE > X
               OVULE = OVULE + 1
            Loop
'Swap value in FRUIT(OVULE) with value in FRUIT(NOL)
            If OVULE <> NOL Then
               HOLD = FRUIT(OVULE)
               FRUIT(OVULE) = FRUIT(NOL)
               FRUIT(NOL) = HOLD
               End If
```

```
            NOL = NOL - 1
            Loop
' FRUIT(1) now already contains the only ovule left

' Count number of carpels with a pair of seeds
         B = 2
         For OVULE = 1 To 10
            If B = 2 Then
               B = 1
            Else
               B = 2
            End If
            If B = 2 Then
               NP = NP + FRUIT(OVULE - 1) * FRUIT(OVULE)
            End If
            Next OVULE
         NFL = NFL - 1
         Loop
'Finished simulating the fruits with R seeds

      Next R
'Finished simulating all the fruits with < 9 seeds

   NP = NP + Worksheets("Sheet1").Cells(9,1) * 4
   NP = NP + Worksheets("Sheet1").Cells(10,1) * 5
'No need to permute the fruits with 9 or all 10

'Finished simulating this data set
'Write the value in NP in row NS of 2nd column of Sheet1

   Worksheets("Sheet1").Cells(NS, 2) = NP

   Next NS
'Finished simulating all the data sets

MsgBox ("End Carpel")
End Sub 'CARPEL
```

2.5   You practice

More about the EXCEL macro editor

To become more comfortable with the EXCEL macro editor, you might like to copy macro CARPEL from Section 2.4 into your EXCEL macro editor. To do this, open a new workbook in EXCEL, pull down the "Tools" menu, open the "Macro" menu and choose "Visual Basic Editor". Pull down the "Insert" menu and click on "Module". Then, click on "Module1" in the "Project" window. Go to the "Properties" window below and rename "Module1" as CARPEL. Now read from Section 2.4, using your keyboard to copy macro "CARPEL" into the macro editor. Now return to EXCEL "Sheet1" and enter in column 1, rows 3 through 10 the numbers of fruits with row seeds, i.e., in row 3 enter the number of fruits with 3 seeds, etc. You can use David's data or just make up some of your own. When you have done this, pull down the file menu and save "Book1.XLS" as "CARPEL.XLS" on the desktop. You can save it away in an appropriate folder when you are finished working on it.

If you are like me, you will make mistakes copying Section 2.4. Some may show up in red (probably) as you copy. You can correct these right away. When you run the macro you have copied, other mistakes may stop the execution, which will return you to the editor with EXCEL's explanation for why it got confused. Look at Section 2.4 to make the corrections. The worst kind of mistake is one that allows the macro to run to completion with no complaints from VBE or EXCEL, but wrong answers appear on the spreadsheet. It is always a good idea to have in mind what constitutes a realistic answer, so you can watch out for ridiculous results. Unfortunately, some wrong answers can look very plausible. We will discuss techniques to deal with this problem later. When CARPEL finishes, column 2 of "Sheet1" should contain 1000 values for the number of carpels with a pair of seeds, which you can ask EXCEL to sort so that you can see an estimate of the predicted probability distribution for the number of carpels with a pair of seeds.

A real exercise problem

Once you are comfortable editing, correcting, saving, etc., you are ready to challenge yourself with the problem below. If you are reading this text in a class situation, it is very good to team up with a classmate to work together. It will help to design on paper spaces in the computer's memory that you will need to hold data, indices, intermediate results, and simulated values of your test statistic. Give these places names that will help you remember what you intend for them to mean. Describe the steps in the calculating process that you envision (the program flow) in a familiar language that is not restricted by the rules of VBE. Finally, open the EXCEL macro editor. Start by naming and typing the spaces in memory that you intend to use. It is good for both you and your team mate to be working together on one computer, one of you typing and the other watching, questioning, and commenting. Remember to be patient with yourselves. After 40 years of experience, my programs rarely run the first time (or the second or the third ...), so do not expect yours to.

One wintry afternoon in Michigan just before dark, Patricia caught 13 Chickadees after a day of foraging for seeds. She weighed each one accurately and released it to find its roost for the night. The next morning just after dawn near the same place she caught 11 Chickadees leaving their roosts. She weighed each one accurately and released it to go spend another day foraging for seeds. One way that Chickadees could avoid freezing during a cold winter's night might be to metabolize fat stores to release energy. If so, they should weigh slightly less in the morning than they do at night. To see if her data support this idea, Patricia wants to test the hypothesis that the birds did not actually lose any weight overnight, i.e., any apparent differences could have happened at random. Her concept, at random, is that any one of the bird weights was just as likely to have been recorded in the evening instead of in the morning, or in the morning instead of in the evening, as any other bird weight. She needs to calculate something relevant from her bird weight data (a test statistic) to test her hypothesis. If it has a value, calculated from her observed data, that is improbably high or low, compared to the probability distribution predicted for it by her hypothesis, then she can reject the hypothesis that her birds do not actually lose weight overnight.

You are challenged to design a test statistic and write a macro to predict a probability distribution for it, to test Patricia's idea that birds lose weight overnight. Notice that, to design a test statistic and write a macro to predict its probability distribution under Patricia's hypothesis, you do not need to know the values of the weights that Patricia measured, but to run your macro you will need to have data. It is useful to invent a small data set for which you can easily calculate by hand values for the purpose of testing your macro, before running it with real data.

You have been given step 1 of this task by the biological context of Patricia's research. Step 2 is to structure the data so that you can ask the question of interest. Think of how you could reserve and name places in the computer's memory to hold Patricia's measurements and information about how many there are and when they were made. Step 3 is to implement Patricia's hypothesis of random, so that you can simulate it to create data sets like hers that would be examples of what might be observed if her hypothesized random process were generating the data. By changing the names of places, you should be able to re-use some of the statements from macro CARPEL to implement the simulation of data sets. Step 4 is to design a test statistic. Usually there are several reasonable possibilities. Think of something you could observe, count, or calculate from Patricia's data that would usually have a larger (or smaller) value if the birds really did lose weight at night, but an intermediate value if any measurement were as likely as any other to have been made in the evening or in the morning. Write 1000 simulated values on your spreadsheet and then ask EXCEL to order them to show the predicted probability distribution for your test statistic.

How to solve it

At this early stage, this task may seem quite challenging for you, especially if you work alone. If you are in a classroom setting, after you have talked things over with your partner, it may be effective to share ideas all around. When you have some ideas, it is best to develop your macro in steps. Make up 24 bird weights; then open EXCEL and write them on a spreadsheet. Decide which 13 you will interpret as the evening measurements and which 11 you will interpret as the morning measurements. Then open VBE, create a new module, give it a name, and in the editor, write statements to name and type an array with 24 places for these measurements, and to name a place for an index for this array. Look in macro CARPEL to see how this was done for the array, FRUIT() and its index OVULE. Now write statements to read bird weights from your spreadsheet into this array. Follow these with statements to write these same bird weights to a different part of your spreadsheet. Stop your macro here (for now) and run it (click the "Run" box at the top of your screen). Return to your spreadsheet (if not already there) to ensure that your macro wrote the birds weights correctly. If not, go back and try to fix the problem. You will be more likely to see what is wrong if there are two of you working together. Do not edit any more statements into your macro until you are sure that this part is working OK. Then put primes in front of the statements that write the weights to your spreadsheet, and save it.

Next compose statements that calculate the value of your test statistic from these weights. It is a good idea to calculate the value of your test statistic first with pencil and paper, to pay attention to what you actually do, and to note its value. Your calculations may have involved adding several numbers. To do this in your macro, you will need a place to put the sum, call it SUM. Start by putting 0 in SUM and continue by adding into SUM each of the numbers you want to add together. For example, you could count the number of ovules that developed into a seed in FRUIT() by adding the places in FRUIT() like this:

```
SUM = 0
For OVULE = 1 To 10
    SUM = SUM + FRUIT(OVULE)
    Next OVULE
    'Now SUM contains the sum of the 10 places in FRUIT()
```

Instruct your macro to write to your spreadsheet the value that it calculated for the test statistic, taking care not to overwrite your data. Stop your macro here, save your spreadsheet, and run your macro. Now return to your spreadsheet and compare the value of the test statistic there to the value you calculated yourself. If they are not the same, first check to make sure that you did not make a mistake with pencil and paper, and then look for the mistakes in your macro. Working in pairs really helps at this stage. When your macro can calculate the test statistic OK, save your spreadsheet.

Now write the statements to simulate a data set. You should be able to re-use some statements from macro CARPEL, changing only the names of places. Instruct your macro to write a simulated data set on your spreadsheet; be sure to choose a place that does not overwrite your data. Stop here, save your spreadsheet and run your macro. Check your spreadsheet to ensure that your macro seems to be simulating a data set OK. Although there are many possible simulated data sets, there are ways in which any given one may seem to be OK. For example, each original weight should appear once. You may want to look at several simulated data sets. When things look OK, put primes before the statements that write a simulated data set to your spreadsheet. Save your spreadsheet.

Now copy the statements to calculate the test statistic below the statements that simulate a data set. You may need to modify them slightly to calculate the test statistic from the simulated data. For example, you may want to put the simulated value of the test statistic in one place and the observed value in another. Instruct your macro to write the simulated value to your spreadsheet. Save your spreadsheet. Run your macro and examine your spreadsheet to see if the simulated value for the test statistic looks OK.

When everything looks good to go, finally enclose the instructions that simulate a data set and calculate a test statistic in a "For .. Next" loop that executes 1000 times. As in macro CARPEL, use index to write a simulated value of the test statistic to the next row in a column of your spreadsheet. Save your spreadsheet and run your macro. Even though it is simulating 1000 data sets, it should run in a few seconds. If it is still running after a minute, press the "Pause/Break" key to stop execution. You should return to your macro editor. In such cases, the problem is likely to be related to things that control program flow. When your macro has finished, your spreadsheet should have a column of 1000 simulated values of the test statistic. Ask EXCEL to order that column; then look down for the observed value of the test statistic. The index of the row where you find it, or the first value larger (or smaller if your arguments depends on a small value for your test statistic) will estimate its realized significance, when divided by 1000.

Remember lawyers

Lawyers collect data that support the hypothesis (the interests of their paying clients) that they want to argue. Unlike lawyers, scientists are paid in prestige by their own universities, professional societies, national granting agencies, the media, and their own egos. In our society, their prestige derives largely from the failure of experimental data to disprove the hypotheses that they have proposed. Thus, data that have been collected by scientists who have in mind their own hypothesis to test can be contaminated by the lawyer effect. On the other hand, scientists who do not have a clear idea of what hypothesis their data are intended to test may collect irrelevant data, or fail to collect relevant data. One way to avoid this methodological dilemma is for one scientist to collect data to test a hypothesis proposed by a different scientist.

A really convincing argument to support a hypothesis can be made when: (1) the hypothesis predicts something that society does not currently believe; (2) the experiment to gather data to test it is carried out by scientists who do not believe that the hypothesis being tested is correct; and (3) still the data collected are consistent with those predictions. A good example of this is the idea that continents have drifted over the past hundreds of millions of years to the places where they are presently. In the first half of the twentieth century, many people thought this idea was patent nonsense. At great expense, ocean ships were outfitted to make careful measurements of the sea floor, to gather data that would put this silly idea to rest. But no! The data gathered indicated that continents had drifted. Because the scientists designing the experiments and gathering the data were trying hard to disprove the hypothesis, their failure to do so made a stronger argument in favor of continental drift. Of course, as with any statistical argument, each of us has to decide how plausible it might be. Hopefully, our society will improve its ability to appreciate scientists for the methods they use to test hypotheses, whether or not those hypotheses turn out to be consistent with data.

In consideration of these things, it will be instructive for you to write your macro without Patricia's real data. When you have your concepts defined and your program running, make up three different possible data sets. With one, try to imagine data that would be evidence for the idea that birds lost weight overnight. With another, try to imagine data that would be evidence for the idea that birds did not lose weight overnight. With the last, try to imagine data that would leave this question ambiguous. Then run your macro with each data set, and discover the realized significance of the test statistic in each case.

If this problem seems a little overwhelming for you now, do not despair. Just go on to read and work with the example of Section 2.4. Then come back and try again.

3 | Choosing a test statistic

3.1 Significance of what

Data from fossil marine organisms

Raup and Sepkoski (1984a) published a study of the fossils of several hundred marine organisms that lived between about 300 million years ago and about 10 million years ago. They divided this time period into 43 stages of about seven and a half million years each. In each stage they counted the number of taxonomic families that made their last appearance in that stage (presuming that these families went extinct during that stage). Then they compared each pair of successive stages to determine if, from the earlier stage to its next later stage, the number of extinctions went up (U) or down (D). These are their observations:

UU DU DDDU DUUU DU DU DUU DDU DDUU DDDUU DDUUU DDUU DD

Each letter stands for a pair of successive stages. With 43 stages there are 42 pairs of successive stages, and hence 42 letters. An extinction peak occurred whenever a U was followed by a D. Observe that the lengths of the times, in units of stages, of inter-peak intervals are 2, 4, 4, 2, 2, 3, 3, 4, 5, 5, 4. The initial UU is not counted as an inter-peak interval because you cannot be sure when it began. Likewise, the final DD is not counted as an inter-peak interval because you cannot be sure when it ended. The average length of inter-peak interval is about 3 1/2 stages, which in units of years is about 26 MY. One group of scientists suggested that during this 290 MY period, the extinction rate of marine families had risen and fallen periodically, with a period of about 26 MY.

The controversy

A second group of scientists questioned whether the data support this hypothesis. They observed that half the pairs of successive stages showed an increase in extinction rate and half showed a decrease (there are 21 Us and 21 Ds) and so they hypothesized that with probability 1/2 the next successive stage shows an increase in extinction rate, and with probability 1/2 it shows a decrease. This hypothesis implies a non-periodic random process. They showed mathematically that this hypothesis predicts that the average inter-peak interval length approaches 4.0 as the sequence of Us and Ds becomes very long. They argued that this is close enough to the observed average of 3 1/2 to interpret the data as consistent with this hypothesized non-periodic random process.

The first group of scientists replied by asserting that the exact pattern shown in the data would occur only about three times in 100 000 if it were produced by this hypothesized non-periodic process; therefore this non-periodic process should be rejected as a possible explanation of the data. The scientists involved in this controversy published their arguments in *Nature*, 29 May 1986, pp 533–536. Both groups of scientists used the same data, structured in the same way, and the same hypothesized random-data-generating mechanism, but reached opposite conclusions. How could this happen?

Relevance of precision

The two groups of scientists differed in the precision with which they determined a realized significance; the first group calculated a realized significance with great precision, while the second group claimed that 3 1/2 is pretty close to 4. But this does not explain their disagreement. In fact, this difference in precision is appropriate. When arguing to reject a hypothesis, it is quite important to predict a probability distribution (especially its tails) accurately so that you can argue that the observed value of the test statistic is so low (or so high) compared to what the hypothesis predicts that the hypothesis seems unlikely to be an adequate explanation for the data. When arguing that the data are consistent with the hypothesis, any realized significance in the middle 2/3 of a predicted distribution is sufficient.

Could one or both groups have made mathematical mistakes when calculating such different realized significances? I think this is unlikely because my own calculations produced results similar to theirs. When I wrote a program to estimate the probability distribution for the mean inter-peak interval length of 11 intervals, 4 was about the middle and 3 1/2 was near it, as claimed. When I calculated the probability of the pattern shown in the data, I got a very small number, as claimed.

Two irrelevant statistics

The significances argued by the two groups of scientists differ because they are the significances of different test statistics. The first group of scientists replied to the challenge of the second group by accurately calculating the probability of the exact pattern of the data. Any particular exact pattern of data usually occurs with low probability under any hypothesis. It may be useful to calculate the probability of the exact pattern of the data when two or more hypotheses are being compared; the hypothesis under which the probability of the exact pattern of the data is maximum is considered the hypothesis most consistent with the data. This style of argument is called maximum likelihood; it is one of the argument styles mentioned earlier, but not discussed in very much depth in this book. However, when testing a single hypothesis, the exact pattern of the data rarely captures a relevant notion of what is to be explained.

With a simple example, let me clarify the concept of relevant notion. Suppose you toss a coin 100 times to see if it seems fair, i.e., equally likely to come up heads as tails, and get 45 heads and 55 tails. Without actually calculating any probabilities, you think it is probably fair because you did not get too many heads or too many tails. In fact, according to the probability distribution predicted by the hypothesis that the coin is fair, the probability of 45 or fewer heads is between 1/5 and 1/6, which most would consider too probable to reject the hypothesis. On the other hand, given this hypothesis the probability of exactly 45 heads is slightly less than 1/20, which many scientists would consider improbable enough to reject the hypothesis. However, it would be a mistake to reject the hypothesis that the coin is fair based on the probability of exactly 45 heads and 55 tails because this is not the probability of a relevant notion of not too many.

Average inter-peak interval length is another example of a test statistic irrelevant to the hypothesis in question. Average inter-peak interval length might be a reasonable estimate for the period, if the process were periodic. However, the question is not, what is the period?, but rather, is the process periodic?. A periodic process has nearly the same length each period. The average length of a period fails to capture this notion. The failure of an irrelevant test statistic to differ significantly from the value predicted for it is irrelevant to scientific argument.

Relevant statistics

To test the plausibility of the same simple, non-periodic explanation for the data hypothesized by both groups, you need a test statistic that measures something that would differ between a periodic and a non-periodic variation in extinction rates. An appropriate test statistic would measure the variability in the length of the period, because period length might vary less in a periodic process than in a non-periodic process. You come to know this by first understanding the role that a test statistic plays in scientific argument, and then paying close attention to the question you are trying to test with argument and data. You need to ensure that the test statistic represents something about the hypothesized explanation that is relevant to what is being questioned and argued, and that the probability distribution for that relevant statistic is accurately predicted so you can use it to determine its significance realized by the data.

Freedom to choose any statistic

Before the recent advent of copious computing power, you would not have been able conveniently to calculate predicted probability distributions for just any test statistic. Instead, at great computational cost, a few standard probability distributions were calculated so that their percentiles could be published in books. A few cleverly pre-structured hypotheses would predict these pre-calculated probability distributions for a few cleverly pre-constructed test statistics. If you could use these hypotheses and test statistics, then you could look up their realized significances in the books where the percentiles of the predicted distributions were published. Understandably, the clever mathematics involved in all of this was not well understood by most good scientists, and so the statistical steps in scientific argument were handed over to statistical specialists, many of whom, although good statisticians, did not fully understand the science of the scientists they were trying to help. By contrast, today with a small time investment in what is essentially a language skill, you can learn to program your computer to calculate predicted distributions for any test statistic you can define. This investment by itself will not prevent you from defining and using irrelevant test statistics. However, it will give you the opportunity to define and use simple, direct, relevant test statistics, unencumbered by much need for specialized mathematical knowledge, or the constraints of classical statistics, once you have mastered the art of recognizing them.

3.2   Implement the program

Here I finalize the details of a hypothesis and test statistic that capture the spirit of the periodicity controversy raised by Raup and Sepkoski (1984b). Then I design and implement a computer program (macro) that calculates the realized significance of the observed value of that test statistic according to the probability distribution predicted by that hypothesis.

Hypotheses of non-periodicity

I need to formulate a specific hypothesis that the observed row of ups and downs was not influenced by factors that would make the lengths between successive occurrences of U followed by D be nearly equal, i.e., seem periodic. If the observed sequence of ups and downs were typical in some essential way of what a non-periodic hypothesis predicts, then there would be little reason to believe that outside factors to produce periodicity were at work. If the observed data were atypical of what a non-periodic hypothesis predicts because there was too little variability in inter-peak distance, then I could argue that outside factors seem to have been operating to produce periodicity in extinction rate.

There are many reasonable ways to define explicit random-data-generating mechanisms that embrace the notion of non-periodic, i.e., no influences that reduce variability of inter-peak lengths. One simple way is to hypothesize that, in any subsequent stage, the extinction rate could increase or decrease with equal probability; $Pr(up) = Pr(down) = 1/2$. This is the hypothesis used in the arguments of each of the two groups of contending scientists. However, I chose a different hypothesis, for reasons explained below.

Other considerations being equal, I can make a stronger statistical argument with a hypothesis that simulates a data set that resembles the observed data set in ways that are not in question, and varies from the observed data set only in ways that are in question. For example, whether or not there are 43 stages is NOT in question. The expected value of inter-peak distance is 4 (the value used in the argument of the second group of scientists) only if there is a very large number of stages; for 43 stages its value is slightly less than 4 because very long inter-peak distances are not possible. The second group of scientists implicitly hypothesized data sets with substantially more than 43 stages. A statistical argument based on a hypothesis that included possible data sets with fewer or more stages would not be so convincing as one based on a hypothesis that only considered data sets with 43 stages, just like the observed data. Even more convincing would be an argument based on a hypothesis that simulated 43 stages with 21 ups and 21 downs, just as was observed, because the number of ups and downs is not in question either. Thus, I use the hypothesis that all arrangements of the 21 ups and the 21 downs are equally likely.

Computational overview

To put in motion a random-data-generating mechanism that chooses any rearrangement equiprobably, first I name and type a place, UOD(45), in the computer's memory to hold the array of ups and downs, and an index to read it. On my EXCEL "Sheet3" I have entered, in the first 42 rows of column 1, the observed sequence of ups and downs, entering 1 for up and 0 for down. My macro read the sequence into UOD() like this.

```
Dim UOD(42) As Byte
    'up or down, the 42 boundaries between
    'pairs of successive stages: 1=up 0=down
Dim R As Integer
    'to read and write row R of the worksheet
For R = 1 To 42
UOD(R) = Worksheets("Sheet3").Cells(R,1)
Next R
```

Now that my macro has statements that read the observed data from a worksheet into the computer's memory, my macro continues with statements that calculate the value of the test statistic for the observed data. Then it simulates 1000 data sets using the hypothesis that any sequential arrangement of the 21 ups and 21 downs is equally likely. For each simulated data set, my macro uses the same statements to calculate the value of the test statistic for simulated data as it did to calculate its value for observed data. I leave the details of how to calculate the test statistic for later in this section.

Sample the chosen hypothesis with computation

My macro chooses a rearrangement of UOD() equiprobably from among all possible, in the same way that macro CARPEL rearranged FRUIT(). First choose equiprobably one of the 42 places in UOD(); if it is not the last place then swap the contents of that place with the contents of the last place. Then choose equiprobably one of the first 41 places in UOD(); if it is not the 41st place then swap its contents with those of the 41st place. Continue like this until only the first place is left. Instructions look like this:

```
Randomize 'Initialize the random number generator
NL = 42 'Number of un-chosen places left in UOD()
For K = 1 To 41 'Choose a random place to swap 41 times
    X = Rnd * NL 'Choose a random number 0.0 < X < NL
    J = 1      'Find the smallest Integer J larger than X
    Do Until J > X 'to use an index for UOD
        J = J + 1
    Loop
    If J <> NL Then
        HOLD = UOD(J) 'Use J to index UOD() and swap
        UOD(J) = UOD(NL) 'with last unchosen place
        UOD(NL) = HOLD
    End If
    NL = NL - 1 'Decrement NL
Next K
```

Choosing a permutation equiprobably is a simple random-data-generating mechanism that is commonly used in hypotheses like the one here in which we suppose that no outside influences are making some possible arrangements more or less likely than others. This same concept of equiprobable permutations was used to generate data under the fruit-mediated mechanisms described earlier in the study of *Amelanchier arborea*. The algorithm encoded above has been known and used by many for years; it did not originate in this book or with me. I will use this algorithm again in other examples.

Calculate a relevant statistic

Now that I have written statements to read a data structure and implement a random-data-generating process, I still need to determine exactly how to calculate something that indicates how variable are the inter-peak lengths in any row of ups and downs. There are several reasonable ways to make this notion precise. In this example I will use a variance-like test statistic: the average squared difference between the inter-peak lengths and their mean. To calculate this, I named spaces in the computer's memory, like this:

```
Dim IPLEN(25) As Single 'inter-peak interval lengths
Dim NOI As Byte          'number of such lengths
Dim B As Byte            'UOD index
Dim P As Byte            'P = previous peak index
```

Discover inter-peak intervals

Now I need statements to discover the inter-peak intervals and how long they are. A peak occurs when 1 is followed by 0, so I use this test sentence in an "If .. Next" statement: (UOD(B) = 1) And (UOD(B + 1) = 0)

These instructions discover inter-peak lengths:

```
NOI = 0   'no intervals found yet
P = 0     'no peak found yet
B = 0     'start before first stage boundary
Do Until B = 41
   B = B + 1 'test for a peak
   If (UOD(B) = 1) And (UOD(B + 1) = 0) Then
      If P > 0 Then 'found next peak
         NOI = NOI + 1
         IPLEN(NOI) = B - P
      End If 'P done with this interval or 1st partial
      P = B
   End If ' (U done with this peak, or no peak found
Loop 'B = finished Do Until looking at all 42 Us or Ds
```

After my macro finds the first peak, for each subsequent peak it increments NOI, subtracts the previous peak index P from the current peak index B to calculate inter-peak length, and stores in IPLEN(NOI). These inter-peak lengths can now be used to calculate the mean inter-peak length and then the test statistic, the average squared difference between an inter-peak length and that mean.

These instructions are a little tricky, so I will explain them again in more detail. The outer "Do Until B = 41 .. Loop" moves the boundary index, B, along so that each pair of successive boundaries is considered in turn. Each boundary is tested for peak status as described above. If no peak is found, then the next pair of boundaries is examined. When a peak is found, an "If .. Next" tests to see if it is the first peak or a subsequent peak. The first peak is indicated by a 0 in place P. When a subsequent peak is found, its location is in B, so the inter-peak interval length is revealed by B − P. Then the contents of B are put into P so that, when the next peak is found, P contains the index of the previous peak.

"Do Until" is followed by an expression that is either true or false; while it is true, the statements on all the lines below it, down to the line "Loop", are repeatedly executed. In this case, there are two statements between the "Do Until" and the "Loop". The first increments B. The second is a single "If" statement with many lines. It too contains an expression that is either true or false but, unlike the "Do Until" statement, the statement(s) following the "Then" is (are) executed only once. In this case, there is only one statement following the "Then"; it is another "If" statement with many lines. When "Do Until" "or "If" statements have many lines, it is good practice to insert a comment after their "Loop" of "End If" that repeats the first few characters following the "Do Until" or "If"; this shows which "Do Until" or "If" you intend to be ending.

Finally, these statements are repeated 1000 times to simulate 1000 sample values for the test statistic. My macro writes these to a column of a spread-sheet. After the macro runs, they are sorted to estimate the test statistic's probability distribution predicted by the hypothesis that any sequence of 21 ups and 21 downs is equally likely.

Testing the macro

While writing my macro, I used the following statements to ensure that it is discovering interval lengths correctly:

```
For R = 1 To 42
        Worksheets("Sheet3").Cells(R,4) = UOD(R)
    Next R
For R = 1 To NOI
    Worksheets("Sheet3").Cells(R,5) = IPLEN(R)
    Next R
```

Initially, my macro stopped here. I saved it. Then I ran it. Then I looked at "Sheet3" to see in the 4th column a random permutation of the ups and downs. I looked down this column, noting the lengths of the inter-peak intervals and comparing them to what my macro had written in column 5. If the inter-peak intervals were not correct, I would know that I still had mistakes to correct in my macro. I would make changes and re-run my macro until it could get this right. Then I put primes before the statements that write on the spreadsheet so that they will not execute when I continue to develop my macro. I can easily remove them if I need to check this part again.

When my macro was able to discover inter-peak interval lengths, I continued with statements to use them to calculate mean interval length and mean squared differences.

The first three statements appear at the beginning of my macro.

```
Dim MIL As Single    'mean interval length
Dim MSD As Single    'mean squared difference
Dim IX As Byte       'internal index for IPLEN()
```

The following statements appear after discovering interval lengths.

```
MIL = 0              'initialize mean interval length
For IX = 1 To NOI    'add the interval lengths into MIL
    MIL = MIL + IPLEN(IX)
    Next IX          'done adding interval lengths into MIL
MIL = MIL / NOI      'replace MIL with mean interval length
MSD = 0              'initialize mean squared difference
For IX = 1 To NOI    'add sum of squared differences in MSD
    MSD = MSD + (IPLEN(IX) - MIL) * (IPLEN(IX) - MIL)
    Next IX 'done For IX accumulating squared differences
```

```
MSD = MSD / NOI 'replace MSD with its average
Worksheets ("Sheet3").Cells(1, 2) = MIL * 1000
Worksheets ("Sheet3").Cells(2, 2) = MSD * 1000
```

After these statements execute, MSD contains the observed value of the test statistic, the Mean of the Squared Difference of interval length from average interval length. When composing my macro, I stopped here, saved it, and ran it. Then I looked in cells (1,2) and (2,2) to ensure that it calculated the same values for MIL and MSD that I had calculated by hand. If not, I would go back to the macro editor to look for mistakes and correct them until it gets them right.

Now that my macro can calculate the value of the test statistic for the observed data, I will reuse almost the same statements to calculate in SMSD the value of the test statistic for simulated data. In the rare cases where, in a simulated data set, there is only 1 or 0 instance of U followed by D in a random re-arrangement, there are no intervals and NOI contains 0. You cannot divide by 0 so my macro leaves MIL at 0 and puts 43.0 into SMSD, as a flag.

Estimate realized significance

The realized significance that the observed value of the test statistic in MSD is surprisingly low is the probability that a sample from the probability distribution predicted for the test statistic by the hypothesis is equal to, or less than, the observed value in MSD. My macro samples the predicted probability distribution by using the hypothesis to simulate a random data set and then calculating in SMSD a value for the test statistic using that simulated data set. My macro simulates 1000 such samples and increments a significance counter, which I call SIGLO, each time a simulated value is less than or equal to the observed value. SIGLO divided by 1000 approximates the realized significance of the observed value. If that fraction is small, e.g., < 50/1000, then the observed interval lengths vary too little to have been generated as if by the hypothesized data-generating mechanism. It increments another significance counter, which I call SIGHI, each time a simulated value is greater than or equal to the observed value.

For each of 1000 simulated data sets, counted in NSIM, my macro calculates a value for SMDS and writes it in the third column of "Sheet3". It then compares it to the value in MSD and increments the significance counters as appropriate. At the beginning of my macro, I named and typed as Integer the places NSIM, SIGLO, and SIGHI. Finally, the statements that manipulate the contents of places look like this:

```
SIGHI = 0
SIGLO = 0
Randomize
For NSIM = 1 To 1000
    Statements to simulate a data set and calculate MSD
    Worksheets("Sheet3").Cells(NSIM,3) = MSD * 1000
'Write current simulated value of MSD in row NSIM column 3
    If SMSD >= MSD Then SIGHI = SIGHI + 1
    If SMSD <= MSD Then SIGLO = SIGLO + 1
    Next NSIM
'Done simulating 1000 data sets
Worksheets("Sheet3").Cells(1,5) = SIGLO
Worksheets("Sheet3").Cells(2,5) = SIGHI
```

After my macro has run, on Worksheet 3 the second row of the second column will contain the observed value (times 1000) of the test statistic and the third column will contain 1000 sampled values of the test statistic. As with the example of Chapter 2, you can ask EXCEL to sort the 1000 sampled values with smallest on top. Then scan down the sorted column to find the first value that is greater than the observed value. Its row index minus one should be the same as the value of SIGLO in the first row of the fifth column. Divided by 1000, this is the realized significance that the observed value of the test statistic is too low.

Using significance to argue

The controversy in question in this example is whether or not the value in MSD is low enough to enable an argument that, through ancient times, the extinction rate of marine families was periodic. If the observed measure of the variability of inter-peak intervals is unusually low given the hypothesis above (representing a concept that the process is NOT periodic), then random samples of the probability distribution predicted by that hypothesis will rarely be less than or equal to the observed value, so that the realized significance will be a small value. For example, if the observed value of the test statistic exceeded, or was equal to, only the smallest (first) 50 samples in sorted column 3, then the realized significance would be $p = 0.05$. The larger the value of the realized significance, the weaker the argument (based on this hypothesis and statistic) that extinction rate varied periodically. Although in this example it is not an issue, in general, the observed value of a test statistic could possibly be unusually high, which in other cases might be relevant to the statistical argument. The realized significance that the test statistic is high is shown in SIGHI.

Statements comprising my entire EXCEL macro are shown in the next section as Sub PERIOD().

3.3   Sub PERIOD

```
Sub PERIOD()

'Period reads observed U's and D's from column 1, rows 1 .. 42
'of Sheet3. Discovers the inter-peak intervals

'Calculates in MIL mean interval length, and then in MSD
'mean squared difference between MIL and the observed
'length. MSD is the test statistic

'1000 data sets are simulated under the hypothesis that the
'21 Us and 21 Ds could have occurred in any order with equal
'probability. For each, simulated mean squared difference
'is calculated in SMSD to estimate the probability
'distribution for MSD predicted by this hypothesis

'Begin block to structure computer's memory

Dim UOD(42) As Byte
'42 boundaries between pairs of successive stages,
'1=up 0=down
Dim R As Integer
'to read and write row R of the worksheet

Dim IPLEN(25) As Single
'Inter-Peak interval Lengths
```

```
Dim NOI, B, P, IX As Byte
'for discovering lengths of intervals:
'# of intervals, last peak index, peak index, interval index

Dim MIL, MSD, SMSD As Single
'mean interval length, mean squared difference,
'simulated mean squared difference

Dim X As Single 'to sample random number generator

Dim J, K, NL As Integer
'for permuting: random index, next place, number left

Dim HOLD As Byte 'to switch places during permuting

Dim NSIM, SIGHI, SIGLO As Integer
'for counting simulations and realized significances

'Begin block to manipulate data structures

MsgBox ("Begin PERIOD")
For R = 1 To 42
   UOD(R) = Worksheets("Sheet3").Cells(R, 1)
   Next R
'done reading observed data

NOI = 0 'no intervals found yet
P = 0 'no peak found yet
B = 0 'start before first stage boundary

Do Until B = 41
   B = B + 1
   If (UOD(B) = 1) And (UOD(B + 1) = 0) Then 'found a peak
      If P > 0 Then 'found an interval
         NOI = NOI + 1
         IPLEN(NOI) = B - P
         End If
      'done processing this non-first interval
```

```
    P = B
    End If 'done considering this peak or no peak found

  Loop 'B = 41
'finished Do Until looking at all 42 boundaries

For R = 1 To NOI
    Worksheets("Sheet3").Cells(R, 4) = IPLEN(R)
    Next R

'The above 3 statements show whether this macro is discovering
'interval lengths correctly in the observed data
'You can cut and paste them into the simulation loop to test
'there, but just simulate one data set at a time
'Then precede them with prime so that they do not compile
'and execute when you simulate 1000 times

MIL = 0 'initialize mean interval length
For I = 1 To NOI 'accumulate in MIL sum of interval lengths
    MIL = MIL + IPLEN(I)
    Next I
'done For I accumulating IPLEN

MIL = MIL / NOI 'replace MIL with its average

Worksheets("Sheet3").Cells(1, 2) = MIL * 1000

MSD = 0 'initialize mean absolute difference
For I = 1 To NOI 'accumulate in MSD sum of squared differences
    MSD = MSD + (IPLEN(I) - MIL) * (IPLEN(I) - MIL)
    Next I
'done For I accumulating squared differences
MSD = MSD / NOI 'replace contents of MSD with its average

Worksheets("Sheet3"). Cells(2, 2) = MSD * 1000
'Write test statistic (* 1000 to increase printed precision)
```

```
SIGHI = 0

SIGLO = 0 'Initialize significance counters

Randomize
For NSIM = 1 To 1000 'Simulate 1000 data sets
        'permute UOD using the same algorithm as in Sub CARPEL
        NL = 42
        For K = 1 To 41
            X = Rnd * NL
            J = 1
            Do Until J > X
                   J = J + 1
                   Loop
            If J <> NL Then 'switch contents of UOD(J) and UOD(NL)
                   HOLD = UOD(J)
                   UOD(J) = UOD(NL)
                   UOD(NL) = HOLD
                   End If
            NL = NL - 1
            Next K


'           For J = 1 To 42
'           Worksheets("Sheet3").Cells(J, 5) = UOD(J)
'           Next J


'While writing your macro, these statements show whether it is
'permuting UOD OK. Use primes to remove them when macro runs

'Reuse statements above to find inter-peak lengths
   NOI = 0 'no intervals found yet
   P = 0 'no peak found yet
   B = 0 'start before first stage boundary

Do Until B = 41
   B = B + 1
   If (UOD(B) = 1) And (UOD(B + 1) = 0) Then 'found a peak

     If P <> 0 Then 'found an interval
         NOI = NOI + 1
```

```
            IPLEN(NOI) = B - P
            End If 'done processing this interval


        P = B
        End If 'done considering this peak or no peak found


Loop 'B = 41
'finished Do Until looking at all 42 boundaries


'For R = 1 To NOI
' Worksheets("Sheet3").Cells(R, 4) = IPLEN(R)
' Next R


'Execute these statements while testing your macro to see that
'it is discovering inter-peak lengths in permuted data sets OK


MIL = 0 'initialize mean interval length
If NOI > 0 Then 'in very rare cases there will be no intervals
    For I = 1 To NOI 'accumulate in MIL sum of interval lengths
        MIL = MIL + IPLEN(I)
        Next I
    'done accumulating

    MIL = MIL / NOI 'replace contents of MIL with its average

    SMSD = 0 'initialize simulated mean squared difference
    For I = 1 To NOI 'accumulate in SMSD simulated MSD
        SMSD = SMSD + (IPLEN(I) - MIL) * (IPLEN(I) - MIL)
        Next I
    SMSD = SMSD / NOI 'replace contents of SMSD with its average
    End If 'NOI
'done calculating simulated value of test statistic
    If MIL = 0 Then SMSD = 43
        'In the very rare case that there are no intervals,
        'load SMSD with a large flag value


Worksheets("Sheet3").Cells(NSIM, 3) = SMSD * 1000
        'Write simulated value of test statistic in column 3
```

```
    If MSD <= SMSD THEN SIGHI = SIGHI + 1
    If MSD >= SMSD THEN SIGLO = SIGLO + 1

    Next NSIM
'done 1000 simulated data sets
Worksheets("Sheet3").Cells(1,5) = SIGLO
Worksheets("Sheet3").Cells(2,5) = SIGHI

MsgBox ("Sub PERIOD has finished")
End Sub
```

4 | Random variables and distributions

4.1 Random variables

At random

We use the term, at random, in everyday speech, where it has a vague, intuitive meaning, but in order to use the term, at random, to make statistical arguments explicit, it must be clearly defined. There are philosophical debates and different schools of thought to define what, at random, should mean, especially as it applies to natural phenomena whose behavior we cannot predict with much precision from known deterministic causes. Although we may not be able to predict measurable values with much precision, usually there are some constraints and some patterns. If some quantitative aspect of a phenomenon is observed many different times, its values may tend to fall in a given range with an approximate frequency. One school of thought, called the frequentists, define the term, at random, in this way: something observed under specified natural conditions varies at random if, when large numbers of values are observed independently, they tend to fall in specified ranges with consistent frequencies. I will not discuss other schools of thought here, but for purposes of reading this text, you can consider yourself a frequentist.

The frequentist concept can be idealized to enable us to say, in some cases, what we think those frequencies should be. For example, flipping a coin results in two possible observations: heads or tails. We say that the coin is fair if the frequency of each of those two values is approximately 1/2 when the coin is flipped independently a large number of times. For our purposes generally, the words, observations are made independently, mean that if we observe the value of a flip, it does not affect the frequencies of the values of subsequent flips. More generally, "observations are made independently" means that if we know the observed value of an instance of a random process, then it does not change the frequencies with which possible values will be observed in a subsequent instance.

Random process

Rolling a die lets us observe one of its six sides. The die is fair means that, if the die is rolled many times, the frequency of observing any given side tends to be 1/6. Flipping and rolling are examples of random processes from which a value can be observed. The values in these examples are qualitative states: heads or tails, and patterns of dots. The examples in the opening chapters are random processes that can assume one of several qualitative states: possible arrangements of ovules that ripened into seeds among the five carpels; and possible arrangements of ups and downs in rates of extinction of families of marine animals. In both of these examples, the probability distribution of the random process assigns equal probability to each possible state. Such distributions are called, equiprobable. Random processes need not have equiprobable distributions.

Some random processes determine states with numerical values. Such states may inherit some of the arithmetic properties of numbers: we might be able to say that one state is bigger than another; or that one state is three times bigger than another; or that a state is above or below the average value, etc. For example, the random process that flipped a fair coin five times could determine a value that was the number of heads; possible values would be 0, 1, 2, 3, 4, 5. Note that the probability distribution for this random process would not be equiprobable.

Continuous distributions

All these examples of random processes can take only a finite number of distinct qualitative states so we can easily describe their probability distributions by specifying the frequency (probability) of each possible state. However, some random processes determine one of a very large number of possible numerical values with decimal points. In such cases, we often describe their probability distributions as if the random process could, in theory, determine any decimal point value in a specified range. Such distributions are called continuous distributions. We cannot specify a probability for each possible value because there are too many, but sometimes we can give a rule that can determine the frequency with which an observed value would fall in any given interval of possible values. The uniform distributions constitute one common family of continuous distributions; they correspond to the equiprobable distributions in the examples above.

A common way to describe a continuous distribution is with its density function. The horizontal axis of the graph of a density function represents the values that the random process can take, and the vertical axis represents their so-called density. To determine the probability that the random process assumes a value in a given range of possible values, we determine the area under the graph of its density function and above the horizontal axis between the limits for the given range of values. Because a random process always assumes one of its possible values, with probability 1.0 (certainty), the value will fall somewhere in the entire range of possible values. Thus, the area under the entire density function is always 1.0. For some density functions, it is easy to calculate the area of a given range. For example, the graph of the density function of the uniform distribution of values between 0.0 and 1.0, denoted as **u**, is the horizontal line between 0.0 and 1.0, and one unit above the horizontal axis, as shown in Figure 4.1. When $0.0 \leq a < b \leq 1.0$, the probability that a sample of a random process with this uniform distribution has a value between a and b is the area between a and b under this horizontal line, simply $b - a$.

Consider a random process with the uniform distribution of possible values between 1.0 and 3.0. We will denote this distribution, **u**[1.0, 3.0]. Visualize its density function as a horizontal line half a unit above the

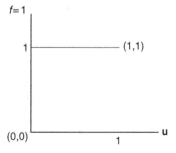

Figure 4.1 Density function f for **u**[0,1], the uniformly distributed random variable with range [0,1].

horizontal axis between 1.0 and 3.0. The probability that a sample of this random process has a value between a and b, with $1.0 \leq a < b \leq 3.0$, is $(b - a) \times 1/2$, because the height of the rectangle under the density function between a and b is now only 1/2.

Many probability density functions are more complicated than this; to calculate the area under them between a given range of possible values requires integral calculus. Some density functions are so complicated that mathematicians cannot calculate this area even using integral calculus. With computation you can estimate these areas, or the probabilities to which they correspond, accurately without using calculus. This is one of the strengths of a computational approach. How to do this is the subject of Section 4.2.

Random variable

When a random process happens and we observe a resulting value of a particular thing, that value is called a sample of the process. The particular thing observed is called a random variable. Thus, the observed value of a random variable is also called a sample of the random variable. Recall that a description of the frequencies of possible values that define a concept of at random is called a probability distribution. We say that a random variable has a specified probability distribution, namely the probability distribution determined by the random process that gives the random variable a value when the process happens. In many cases, once a probability distribution for a random variable has been specified, the mechanics of the random process, and of the random variable observed, do not affect the logic until it is time to re-interpret a statistical argument back into the natural world that we are trying to explain. In such cases, we might call a sample of the random variable simply a sample of its probability distribution. Thus, we have several different ways of talking about a sample, but they all mean basically the same thing.

In most cases, once you have specified the mechanics of a random process specifically enough, you can sample (observe) the value of a random variable determined by an instance of that random process using a computer program (EXCEL macro in our case), without knowing the specific form of the random variable's distribution. How you can do this is the subject of much of the rest of this book.

4.2   Distributions

Computation eliminates calculus

Beginning in the early twentieth century, statisticians have continued to invent random variables, and to describe and manipulate their distributions using calculus. It will be useful for you to develop some appreciation of the theoretical properties of random variables. However, your need to manipulate them using calculus techniques will be virtually eliminated by your ability to approximate their distributions by sampling them a large number of times with a computer.

To describe the distribution of a random variable you ask your computer to sample it a large number of times. One way to see the probability density function estimated by these values is to write them on an EXCEL spreadsheet and use the plotting features of EXCEL to draw graphs for you. I wrote a macro that takes 1000 samples of **u** and writes them on an EXCEL spreadsheet. It looks like this:

```
Dim X As Single
Dim I As Integer
Randomize
For I = 1 To 1000
    X = Rnd
    Worksheets("sheet1").Cells(I,1) = X
    Next I
```

After this macro has run, column 1 will contain 1000 samples of **u**, the uniform distribution between 0.0 and 1.0. Now you can use EXCEL to show you these numbers in various ways. Use EXCEL's sort feature to sort column 1. Samples exceeding 0.1 should start somewhere around row 100, exceeding 0.2 should start around row 200, etc. EXCEL has other features that will show you the shape of the distribution represented by these samples; experiment with them.

Bar graph

You can also write your own macros to reveal the shape of a distribution based on a large number of samples. One way to see a distribution of a random variable is to divide the range of possible values into (say) 10 small equal ranges, and for each sample determine the range in which it falls; then increment a counter for that range. Finally write on an EXCEL spreadsheet the number of times a sampled value falls in each range. This approach makes a bar graph of the frequencies with which samples fall into equal length sub-intervals of the range of possible values.

I took this approach to write a macro to see the distribution of **u**. The range of possible values is from 0.0 to 1.0. I chose 10 sub-intervals, corresponding to 10 bars. More sub-intervals show variation in frequencies at a finer scale, but estimate those frequencies less accurately. To determine the width of each sub-interval, I divided the width of the range of values by the number of sub-intervals; $(1.0 - 0.0)/10 = 0.1$. I named an array SUBIN() of type "Integer" to count the number of samples in each sub-interval. I named and typed some places to use as indices. Then I wrote statements to sample "Rnd" 1000 times, and count the number of samples that fell in each sub-interval. Finally, I wrote statements to write the counts in SUBIN onto a spreadsheet.

Practice writing a macro

Try doing this yourself. Open EXCEL, and VBE. Name a new Module UNIFORM and edit it. Name and Type the places you will need in the computer's memory. Initialize the sub-interval counts equal to 0. Add the instructions to discover the interval in which the next sample falls, and increment the counter for that interval. How to discover the sub-interval in which a sample falls may not be obvious to you. For inspiration, look in Sub CARPEL at the instructions that permute to see how they find an index. Enclose instructions that sample **u** once in a "For ... Next" loop that executes 1000 times. Finally write the counts in SUBIN in a column of a spreadsheet. Often, it is most effective to try to solve programming problems like this one by working in pairs, if possible.

After you have challenged yourself to your satisfaction, look below at my macro UNIFORM. Certainly, your macro will not be exactly like mine; there are usually many ways to write a program to solve a given problem. Some may be more effective than others, and some may be just different. Did your macro have many comments? Did you name and type places you did not really need? Did you find the statements in Sub CARPEL to help you write statements to discover in which sub-interval falls a sample of **u**? Can you find them in my macro below?

```
Sub UNIFORM()
'Displays simulated uniform distribution as a bar graph
MsgBox ("Begin UNIFORM")
Dim SUBIN(10) As Integer
Dim I, J As Integer
Dim X As Single
'Begin Instruction part of macro UNIFORM
For J = 1 To 10 'Initialize sub-interval counters = 0
    SUBIN(J) = 0
    Next J
Randomize 'initialize the random number generator
For I = 1 To 1000 'take 1000 samples of u
    X = Rnd
    Worksheets("Sheet1").Cells(I,1) = X
    'Write sample number I in the first column of Sheet1
    'Discover sub-interval J in which X falls
    X = X * 10 'the integer part of X * 10 is one less than
    J = 1 'the index of the sub-interval in which X falls
    Do Until J > X
        J = J + 1 'increment J until it is one greater than
        Loop 'the integer part of X
    SUBIN(J) = SUBIN(J) + 1 'Increment sub-interval counter
    Next I
    'Done discovering sub-interval for all 1000 samples
For J = 1 To 10
    Worksheets("Sheet1").Cells(J, 3) = SUBIN(J)
    Worksheets("Sheet1").Cells(J, 4) = (J-1) * 0.1
    Worksheets("Sheet1").Cells(J, 5) = J * 0.1
    'In columns 4 and 5 also write the sub-interval limits
    Next J
MsgBox ("End UNIFORM")
End Sub
```

Interpret the bar graph

After macro UNIFORM ran, Columns 3, 4, and 5 of my spreadsheet looked like this. In column 3 are counts of random numbers in sub-intervals; they will change if UNIFORM runs again

Row	Col 3	Col 4	Col 5	Row	Col 3	Col 4	Col 5
1	87	0.0	0.1	6	114	0.5	0.6
2	85	0.1	0.2	7	104	0.6	0.7
3	96	0.2	0.3	8	83	0.7	0.8
4	111	0.3	0.4	9	112	0.8	0.9
5	109	0.4	0.5	10	99	0.9	1.0

In column 4 are the low ends of the sub-intervals; in column 5 the high ends. The way the macro is written, sample values equal to the high end of an interval (it is rare that a sample is equal to anything in particular), are included in that interval. We expect that 1/10 of the samples (100) would fall in each of these 10 intervals. Because **u** was sampled at random, only approximately 100 samples fall in each interval. In this example (the uniform distribution over the range of values from 0.0 to 1.0) an equal number of samples are expected to fall in each interval. You can think of the number of samples in an interval as measuring the average height of the probability density function above the horizontal axis over that interval. In this case, 100 samples equal one unit on the vertical axis. The number of samples in an interval is the height of bar of the bar graph that approximates the probability density function, a horizontal line one unit above the horizontal axis over the range of possible values between 0.0 and 1.0. In general, the bar graphs for probability distributions that are not uniform will have noticeably different numbers of samples in each sub-interval so the heights of the bars will approximate a curve that is not a horizontal line.

You can improve the accuracy of the bar heights by increasing the number of samples. Modify macro UNIFORM, or even better your own macro if you wrote one, to take 10 000 samples. For macro UNIFORM, in the "For I ..." statement you need to change 1000 to 10 000, and you probably want an apostrophe before the statement that writes samples on Sheet1; 10 000 samples is an awful lot of samples to write on a spreadsheet. When I ran macro UNIFORM taking 10 000 samples, I wrote on "Sheet2" so not to overwrite the table on "Sheet1". Columns 2, 3, and 4 of my "Sheet2" looked like this. Of course, if macro UNIFORM ran again, Col 3 would be slightly different.

Row	Col 3	Col 4	Col 5	Row	Col 3	Col 4	Col 5
1	1000	0.0	0.1	6	1043	0.5	0.6
2	982	0.1	0.2	7	986	0.6	0.7
3	980	0.2	0.3	8	961	0.7	0.8
4	1055	0.3	0.4	9	999	0.8	0.9
5	992	0.4	0.5	10	1002	0.9	1.0

With 10 000 samples, 1000 samples represent one unit on the vertical axis. The heights of the bars are now more nearly equal.

Randomize

With 10 000 samples, to help "Rnd" stay more random you should execute procedure, "Randomize", to give it a new seed, every 1000 samples. Below is one possible way:

```
... statements that initialize
For K = 1 To 10
   Randomize
   For I = 1 To 1000
      For I ..
      .. statements in "For I" block
      Next I
   Next K
```

Accuracy vs precision

When the probability density function you seek to approximate with a bar graph is not a horizontal line, you can see the distribution better by using more sub-intervals. If you take the same number of samples, each sub-interval will be represented by fewer samples and so approximate the density function less accurately. Try to modify macro UNIFORM, or your own macro, to take 1000 samples, but count them into 20 sub-intervals. Write your results on "Sheet3". When you have challenged yourself to your satisfaction, look to see how I made the modifications. I changed back "For

I = 1 To 1000". I multiplied X by 20 so that the integer part of $X \times 20$ would be one less than the index of the 20 places in SUBIN(J). I almost forgot to change "Dim SUBIN(20) As Integer" to reserve now 20 places called SUBIN. Finally, when writing columns 4 and 5, I multiplied $(J - 1)$ and J by the new interval width, 0.05. My "Sheet3" is shown below:

Row	Col 3	Col 4	Col 5	Row	Col 3	Col 4	Col 5
1	54	0.00	0.05	11	63	0.50	0.55
2	53	0.05	0.10	12	46	0.55	0.60
3	46	0.10	0.15	13	42	0.60	0.65
4	54	0.15	0.20	14	52	0.65	0.70
5	52	0.20	0.25	15	37	0.70	0.75
6	45	0.25	0.30	16	53	0.75	0.80
7	49	0.30	0.35	17	43	0.80	0.85
8	48	0.35	0.40	18	44	0.85	0.90
9	58	0.40	0.45	19	52	0.90	0.95
10	49	0.45	0.50	20	60	0.95	1.00

Although there are now more sub-intervals, you can see that the heights of the bars are relatively more variable. Fifty is expected in each interval, but counts range from a low of 37 to a high of 64.

These are the results on my "Sheet4" for 10 000 samples.

Row	Col 3	Col 4	Col 5	Row	Col 3	Col 4	Col 5
1	491	0.00	0.05	11	472	0.50	0.55
2	505	0.05	0.10	12	511	0.55	0.60
3	483	0.10	0.15	13	518	0.60	0.65
4	532	0.15	0.20	14	506	0.65	0.70
5	525	0.20	0.25	15	453	0.70	0.75
6	495	0.25	0.30	16	515	0.75	0.80
7	524	0.30	0.35	17	488	0.80	0.85
8	503	0.35	0.40	18	475	0.85	0.90
9	517	0.40	0.45	19	515	0.90	0.95
10	485	0.45	0.50	20	487	0.95	1.00

Here 500 samples are expected in each interval. You can see that the heights of the bars are now more nearly equal.

Pseudo-random

EXCEL VBE provides functions, "Randomize" and "Rnd", that you can use to sample $\mathbf{u}$, the random variable uniformly distributed between 0.0 and 1.0. As you have seen in the previous examples, whenever the function "Rnd" executes, it assumes a value between a and b in the range from $0.0 \le a < b \le 1.0$ with probability very close to $b - a$. Thus, the function, "Rnd", seems to sample the uniform distribution of the random variable $\mathbf{u}$, but it does not actually sample $\mathbf{u}$. There is a large, but only finite, number of different digital configurations in a place of type "Single", so there can be only that finite number of different decimal point numbers stored there. But there is an arbitrarily large number of decimal point numbers in the range, 0.0 to 1.0, so almost all of them cannot be stored in any given place of type "Single"; thus, the probability that "Rnd" will assume any one of their values is 0. However, unless a and b are extremely close to each other, the probability with which "Rnd" chooses a number between a and b will be very close to $b - a$, which is entirely adequate for our purposes.

The next time a statement including "Rnd" executes, "Rnd" seems to assume a value independently of its former value, but it does not quite do so. Because computer programs are necessarily deterministic, so is "Rnd". Each time you reference "Rnd", its algorithm generates deterministically a random number using its previous random number. This is why we call "Rnd" a pseudo-random-number generator. To help make repeated samples made by "Rnd" seem more random, i.e., conform more closely to the concept of independently sampling $\mathbf{u}$ described in the previous section, "Randomize" provides "Rnd" with a different previous random number, called a seed. Often, programs like "Randomize" do this by reading the thousandth-of-a-second state of the computer's time-of-day clock, which changes state so rapidly and independently of what your program is doing that examining its state is like sampling the numbers from 0 to 999 equiprobably. A "Randomize" statement should appear before your first use of "Rnd". To help "Rnd" stay more random, "Randomize" should be executed from time to time to determine a new seed. However, now that computers are so fast, if you execute "Randomize" too frequently, so little time will have gone by that it may discover the same seed and generate the same random numbers over again. I have my macros execute "Randomize" again after "Rnd" has executed several hundred (up to 1000) times.

The computational techniques employed to choose equiprobably a pseudo-random number in a given range can be quite sophisticated and varied. In EXCEL's VBE, some have been implemented for us in the procedures "Randomize" and "Rnd", and we will take it on faith that they work OK. To learn more about random number generators consult Schildt (1986).

4.3   Arithmetic with random variables

Hypotheses make statistics into random variables

You can do arithmetic with random variables. The result is another random variable. When you hypothesize that your observed data are samples of a random process, the test statistic that you calculate, or just observe, from your data becomes a random variable. Its probability distribution is predicted by the hypothesized random process and the structure of your data. In fact, from the point of view of statistical argument, the only relevant thing your hypothesis predicts is the probability distribution for your test statistic. Thus, an important part of understanding statistical argument is understanding what it means to do arithmetic with random variables; this is especially relevant when you take a computational approach to statistical argument.

For example, you can add an ordinary number to a random variable, or you can multiply a random variable by an ordinary number; the result is a new random variable whose probability density function is determined by the probability density function of the random variable involved in the arithmetic, and by the nature of the arithmetic. With practice, you can learn to visualize the probability density function for random variables resulting from some simple arithmetic operations with other random variables. In some cases, there are mathematical techniques to determine the probability density function for random variables that result from more complicated arithmetical operations. Other cases are too complicated even for mathematics to handle. But you do not need to know this mathematics; this book will teach you to estimate by computation the probability density function of ANY random variable calculated from random variables whose distributions you can sample.

Arithmetic with a random variable and numbers

When you do arithmetic with random variables, you must be careful to distinguish between ordinary numbers and samples of random variables. Define the random variable **b** to have one of two possible values, 0 or 1, with distribution $\Pr(\mathbf{b} = 1) = 1/4$, $\Pr(\mathbf{b} = 0) = 3/4$. Suppose you took one sample of **b** and multiplied it by 3, i.e., added it to itself three times. You would get a new random variable with possible values 3 $(= 1+1+1)$ and 0 $(= 0+0+0)$. Denote this new random variable $3 \times \mathbf{b}$. Its distribution is $\Pr(3 \times \mathbf{b} = 3) = 1/4$, $\Pr(3 \times \mathbf{b} = 0) = 3/4$. Now, suppose instead you multiplied **b** times 3 by taking three different samples of **b** and adding them together to make another random variable, denoted **s3**. Its possible values are 0, 1, 2, or 3. Even without determining the distribution of **s3**, we know **s3** must be different from $3 \times \mathbf{b}$ because the possible values of **s3** are not even the same as those of $3 \times \mathbf{b}$.

What is the effect of doing arithmetic with ordinary numbers, as in $3 \times \mathbf{b}$, on the distribution of a random variable? Imagine the distribution of a random variable expressed as a graph of its probability density. Recall that the horizontal axis represents the possible numerical values that the random variable can assume, and the probability that the random variable assumes a value between any two limits on that horizontal axis is equal to the area under the density distribution curve between those two limits. If the random variable can assume only a small, fixed number of possible values, you can think of the density distribution as a bar graph with the bar for each possible value; its height is proportional to the probability of that value. When an ordinary number, c say, is added to a random variable, its distribution curve moves rigidly over the horizontal axis. If c is positive, then it moves c units to the right; if c is negative, then it moves c units to the left. Multiplying a random variable by an ordinary number, c say, stretches or shrinks the distribution curve over the horizontal axis, leaving fixed the point of the curve over the origin. If $c > 1$ then each point of the distribution curve moves away from the vertical axis. If $c < 1$ then each point moves closer to the vertical axis. Each point moves to c times its original distance from the vertical axis.

A macro to convert **u** to another continuous uniform distribution

To apply these concepts, you can use EXCEL to sample a random variable, called **u**[−1.0, 1.0], uniformly distributed between −1.0 and 1.0. You create

u[0.0, 2.0], a random variable uniformly distributed between 0.0 and 2.0, by multiplying **u** by 2, and then add −1.0, like this:

$$\mathbf{u}[-1.0, 1.0] = 2 \times \mathbf{u} - 1.0$$

You can sample **u**[−1.0, 1.0] in an EXCEL macro like this:

$$X = 2 \times \text{Rnd} - 1.0$$

Now X contains a sample of a random variable that assumes a value between a and b, $(-1.0 \le a < b \le 1.0)$ with probability $(b - a)/2$. Although you may be able to envision the probability density function for **u**[−1.0, 1.0], it would be good practice to modify an EXCEL macro from the previous section to report heights of the bars of a bar graph that estimate this density function.

In the case just discussed, only one sample of one random variable is involved; the other numbers are just ordinary numbers. When more than one sample of a random variable, or samples of more than one random variable, are involved in arithmetic, the result is still a new random variable, but its distribution becomes more difficult to determine. In most cases you will need to write an EXCEL macro to estimate it. In some very simple cases, you can determine the distribution for the resulting new random variable by calculating it yourself. It is instructive to examine such a case.

Sum of independent samples of the same binary random variable

Data can often be construed as several independent samples of the same random variable with only two possible values. As above, the binary random variable **b** has two values: 1 or 0. You might think of the values as indicating your success (1) or failure (0) to observe something of interest on an occasion of looking for it. The distribution for **b** can be specified by indicating the probability (often designated by the letter, p) with which **b** assumes the value 1. The only remaining possible value must be assumed with probability, $1 - p$, often designated with the letter, q. We write $\Pr(\mathbf{b} = 1) = p$ and $\Pr(\mathbf{b} = 0) = q$. Because these are only two possible values, $p + q = 1$.

Distinguish between the random variable **b** and its value **b**[1] on an occasion (called 1) of taking a sample. Suppose you observed **b** on three successive occasions (called 1, 2, and 3), to get the numbers **b**[1], **b**[2], and

b[3]. How many 1s (successes) did you observe? To answer this question, you define another random variable to count them. One way you can define a random variable is to describe how to sample it. For example:

$$s3[1] \: != \mathbf{b}[1] + \mathbf{b}[2] + \mathbf{b}[3]$$

To sample **s3** once you need to sample **b** three times and add them together. Here and throughout, I use != to indicate that the equality is by definition, not by logical consequence.

When you sample **b** in such a way that knowledge of the results of any of the samplings does not change the probabilities of the possible results of any of the other samplings, the samples of the random variable **b** are said to be independent. Independence allows you to multiply probabilities to calculate the probability of joint occurrence. Using this principle, you can calculate the distribution for the possible values of **s3**, which are 3, 2, 1, or 0, in the case where $p = 1/4$ (for example) like this:

$$\Pr(\mathbf{s3} = 3) = \Pr(\mathbf{b}[1] = 1) \times \Pr(\mathbf{b}[2] = 1) \times \Pr(\mathbf{b}[3] = 1) \qquad = 1/64$$

$$
\begin{aligned}
\Pr(\mathbf{s3} = 2) = \; &\Pr(\mathbf{b}[1] = 1) \times \Pr(\mathbf{b}[2] = 1) \times \Pr(\mathbf{b}[3] = 0) + \\
&\Pr(\mathbf{b}[1] = 1) \times \Pr(\mathbf{b}[2] = 0) \times \Pr(\mathbf{b}[3] = 1) + \\
&\Pr(\mathbf{b}[1] = 0) \times \Pr(\mathbf{b}[2] = 1) \times \Pr(\mathbf{b}[3] = 1) \qquad = 9/64
\end{aligned}
$$

$$
\begin{aligned}
\Pr(\mathbf{s3} = 1) = \; &\Pr(\mathbf{b}[1] = 1) \times \Pr(\mathbf{b}[2] = 0) \times \Pr(\mathbf{b}[3] = 0) + \\
&\Pr(\mathbf{b}[1] = 0) \times \Pr(\mathbf{b}[2] = 0) \times \Pr(\mathbf{b}[3] = 1) + \\
&\Pr(\mathbf{b}[1] = 0) \times \Pr(\mathbf{b}[2] = 1) \times \Pr(\mathbf{b}[3] = 0) \qquad = 27/64
\end{aligned}
$$

$$\Pr(\mathbf{s3} = 0) = \Pr(\mathbf{b}[1] = 0) \times \Pr(\mathbf{b}[2] = 0) \times \Pr(\mathbf{b}[3] = 0) \qquad = 27/64$$

This distribution is given by the binomial expansion of

$$(1/4 + 3/4)^3 = (1/64 + 9/64 + 27/64 + 27/64) = 1$$

or more generally by the binomial expansion of

$$(p + q)^3 = 1 \times p^3 + 3 \times p^2 \times q^1 + 3 \times p^1 \times q^2 + 1 \times q^3 = 1$$

You can see that the various products of the powers of p and q each represent the probability of one way that the three samples could add up to a particular value of s3. The constants that multiply these products of powers count the number of ways the three samples could add up to the same value, i, for s3. These constants are the number of way you can choose i things from 3. The number of ways does not depend on the value of p, only on the number n of samples. I will use the notation [n,i] to represent the number of ways to choose i things from n.

After n independent trials, the random variable sn counts the number of successful trials: sn[1] != b[1] + b[2] + .. + b[n].

The distribution of sn is given by the expansion of $(p + q)^n$.

Probabilities for possible values of sn are given by its terms:

$$\Pr(sn = i) = p^i \times q^{(n-i)} \times [n, i]$$

Pascal's triangle

Such distributions are called binomial, and the numbers [n,i] are called the binomial coefficients. Although there are computational formulas for the binomial coefficients, one nice way to compute them for small n was invented by the seventeenth-century French mathematician, Pascal. This is the top of Pascal's triangle:

```
1 1
1 2 1
1 3 3 1
1 4 6 4 1
1 5 10 ...
```

The rule is to start the next row with 1, continue with the sum of the number above and the number to its left, and end again with 1. For example, 6 is the sum of the 3 above it and the 3 to the left of that 3. If you name the first column 0, the second 1 and so on, then in row n and column i, you find the binomial coefficient [n,i]. For example row 3 contains the coefficients for s3, no matter what the value of p. For p = 1/3 and q = 2/3, the values 3 2 1 0 of s3 would have the respective probabilities 1/27 6/27 12/27 8/27.

A macro to estimate s3

You can also arithmetically combine continuously varying random variables to make new random variables. For example, define **hat**[1] != **u**[1] + **u**[2], by adding two samples of **u**, the uniformly distributed unit interval discussed earlier. Because such random variables have an infinite number of possible values, you cannot consider all combinations, as you did to calculate the distribution of **s3**. In simple cases like this one, there are calculus techniques to describe the distribution of the new random variable, but with this book you do not need to learn them, so I will not present them. Instead you estimate the distribution by sampling it many times.

You have the tools to estimate a distribution for **hat**. You know the distribution of **s3** for $p = 1/3$. So modify a macro from the previous section to estimate it computationally to see how close you come. You can sample **s3** for $p = 1/3$ in your EXCEL macro like this; initialize the place S3 at 0, then use the fact that Rnd ≤ 0.3333333 is true with probability 1/3 to add 1 to the content of place S3, either 0, 1, 2, or 3 times, to compute a sample of **s3**, like this:

```
S3 = 0;
For I = 1 To 3
    If Rnd <= 0.3333333 Then S3 = S3 + 1
    Next I
```

Of course, these are just the instructions. Your macro will have to name and type I and S3, as well as a table with four places to count frequencies of samples with a given value. Choosing to take 2700 samples as a basis to estimate the distribution allows you to expect convenient round numbers. Here's what I got when I ran my macro:

Value of s3	3	2	1	0
Number of samples	110	609	1199	782
Theoretical number	100	600	1200	800

Use the same approach to write an EXCEL macro to estimate the density distribution for the random variable, **hat**, using 10 sub-intervals. Before you run your macro, try to guess what the distribution will look like. When you get your program to run correctly, sketch the graph of the distribution for **hat** using bar heights your macro writes on a spread-sheet. You can also ask EXCEL to draw a bar graph, or make other drawings, from the individual samples of **hat** you have written on a spreadsheet. Realize that **hat** has a continuous density distribution, which is estimated by counts of samples in discrete sub-intervals. You use the counts in discrete sub-intervals to guess and draw a continuous density distribution. How would you describe the shape of the distribution in words?

Macros to estimate other density distributions

With only slight modifications, you can now write macros to estimate the density distributions for other random variables. Try **u** − **u** (for random variables, this is not 0). Compare **u** × **u** with **u** squared (for random variables, these are not the same). Estimate the probability distribution for **b** × **u**. Why would anyone ever want to sample **b** × **u**? Aaron wanted to. While working on his Ph.D. thesis in archeology studying excavations in ancient Mesopotamia, he observed that a particular stone tool was absent from about half of his excavation sites, but when it was present its abundance seemed equally likely to be any amount from just a little to quite a lot. You never can tell what will be useful, as you continue to think creatively about your science, but with certainty, you cannot use a concept unless you are aware if it.

4.4   Expected value and variance

The middle of a distribution

The distribution of a random variable is commonly described with an indication of its middle and a measure of its width. These two numbers can be used to compare the distribution of one random variable with that of another. They are useful also for inventing or choosing random variables to use in a hypothesized data-generating mechanism or for estimating things. The middle of a distribution of a random variable might be defined as the value that the random variable would exceed with probability 0.5. A major problem with this definition is that there might not be any such value, or there might be many such values. Consider the binary random variable,

b, defined above, with $\Pr(\mathbf{b} = 1) = 1/2$. The probability that **b** assumes a value greater then $1/2$ is $1/2$, but so is the probability that **b** assumes a value greater than any number greater than 0. Next give **b** the distribution $\Pr(\mathbf{b} = 1) = 1/3$. Now there is no number, e, so that $\Pr(\mathbf{b} \ge e) = 0.5$. To get around this, the concept, expected value of a random variable, **r**, written $E(\mathbf{r})$, is defined to be the sum over all its possible values, x, of the products, $x \times \Pr(\mathbf{r} = x)$.

For example, the expected value of **b** with distribution $\Pr(\mathbf{b} = 1) = 1/2$ is calculated like this:

$$E(\mathbf{b}) = 0 \times \Pr(\mathbf{b} = 0) + 1 \times \Pr(\mathbf{b} = 1) = 0 \times 1/2 + 1 \times 1/2 = 1/2$$

or with distribution $\Pr(\mathbf{b} = 1) = 1/3$, like this:

$$E(\mathbf{b}) = 0 \times \Pr(\mathbf{b} = 0) + 1 \times \Pr(\mathbf{b} = 1) = 0 \times 2/3 + 1 \times 1/3 = 1/3.$$

In general, the expected value for **b** is the probability, $\Pr(\mathbf{b} = 1)$.

Because you cannot add up all the possible values of a continuously distributed random variable, its expected value is defined in a different way, but in the same spirit. You multiply the density distribution curve at each point by the corresponding value of the random variable to get a new curve; the expected value is the area under this curve. Calculus can be used to find the area under curves that are not too complicated, but for some very simple curves, you can just look. For example, the density distribution of **u**, the uniformly distributed unit interval, is a horizontal line one unit above the **u** axis. When you multiply it by the corresponding possible values for **u**, the result is a straight line that goes from the origin to $(1,1)$, shown in Figure 4.2. The area of the triangle under this line is $1/2$, i.e., $E(\mathbf{u}) = 1/2$, an intuitively satisfying result. In classical statistics, calculus is used to find the

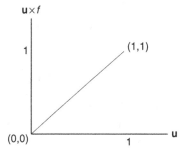

Figure 4.2 The function $f \times \mathbf{u}$. The area under the lower triangle is $\mathrm{Exp}(\mathbf{u}[0,1])$.

expected values of some more complicated continuous distributions, but you do not need calculus to estimate accurately the expected value of any distribution that you can sample with a computer. You can estimate accurately the expected value of a random variable by sampling it many times, adding the samples together, and dividing by the number of samples.

Theoretical properties of expected value

It will be useful to understand more of the theoretical properties of expected value. I will first discuss discrete distributions for which you need only to multiply and to add.

The expected value of **s3** when Pr(**b** = 1) = 1/4 is calculated like this:

$$E(\mathbf{s3}) = 3 \times (1/64) + 2 \times (9/64) + 1 \times (27/64) + 0 \times (27/64) = 48/64 = 3/4$$

Notice that

$$E(\mathbf{s3}) = 3/4 = 1/4 + 1/4 + 1/4 = E(\mathbf{b}) + E(\mathbf{b}) + E(\mathbf{b})$$

In this case, the distribution of the sum of independently sampled random variables has an expected value equal to the sum of the expected values of their distributions. Generally, if **f** and **g** are independent random variables, then

$$E(\mathbf{f} + \mathbf{g}) = E(\mathbf{f}) + E(\mathbf{g}) \tag{4.1}$$

Recall the random variable $3 \times \mathbf{b}$, with possible values 3 and 0, and distribution $\Pr(3 \times \mathbf{b} = 3) = 1/4$, $\Pr(3 \times \mathbf{b} = 0) = 3/4$. Because their possible values are different, so also must be $3 \times \mathbf{b}$ and **s3**. However, the expected values of $3 \times \mathbf{b}$ and **s3** are the same:

$$E(3 \times \mathbf{b}) = 3 \times (1/4) + 0 \times (3/4) = 3/4 = 3 \times E(\mathbf{b}).$$

This suggests that $E(x \times \mathbf{f}) = x \times E(\mathbf{f})$ for any random variable **f** and number x. Recall that $3 \times \mathbf{b}$ means $\mathbf{b}[1] + \mathbf{b}[1] + \mathbf{b}[1]$.

$$E(3 \times \mathbf{b}) = 3/4 = 1/4 + 1/4 + 1/4 = E(\mathbf{b}[1]) + E(\mathbf{b}[1]) + E(\mathbf{b}[1]).$$

Realize that $\mathbf{b}[1]$ and $\mathbf{b}[1]$ are not independent, indeed they are identical. So apparently Equation 4.1 above is true even if **f** and **g** are not independent, and in fact it is. We say, the expected value of the sum is the sum of the expected values. Operations, such as expected value, for which it does not matter whether they operate before or after a sum is taken, are said to be linear operations, also called linear operators or linear functions.

Variance

Variance is a common measure to indicate the spread of the distribution of a random variable. To calculate the variance of a random variable, make a new random variable from the original one by subtracting its own expected value. This slides its distribution horizontally over its value axis so that the expected value of the new random variable is zero. The new random variable indicates how much the old one deviates from its expected value. Now square this new random variable to make another new random variable, which represents the squared deviation of the original random variable from its expected value. The expected value of this new random variable is the variance of the original random variable. Thus variance of a random variable is defined to be the expected value of the squared deviation from its mean. The expected value and the variance of a random variable are numbers, not random variables; they are actually properties of the random variable's distribution.

I will use this definition to calculate the variance of $\mathbf{b}$, with distribution: $Pr(\mathbf{b} = 1) = p$, $Pr(\mathbf{b} = 0) = 1 - p = q$. In the arithmetic below, the symbol $\mathbf{b}$ refers to $\mathbf{b}[1]$, always the same sample of $\mathbf{b}$.

$$V(\mathbf{b}) = E((\mathbf{b} - E(\mathbf{b})) \times (\mathbf{b} - E(\mathbf{b}))) = \text{The definition of } V(\mathbf{b})$$

$$V(\mathbf{b}) = p \times (1 - p) \times (1 - p) + q \times (0 - p) \times (0 - p)$$

$$V(\mathbf{b}) = p \times q \times q + q \times p \times p = p \times q \times (q + p) = p \times q.$$

The variance of $\mathbf{b}$ is the probability of success times the probability of failure.

What happens to variance when you multiply by a number?

$$
\begin{aligned}
\text{Consider } V(5 \times \mathbf{b}) &= E((5 \times \mathbf{b} - E(5 \times \mathbf{b})) \times (5 \times \mathbf{b} - E(5 \times \mathbf{b}))) \\
&= E((5 \times \mathbf{b} - 5 \times E(\mathbf{b})) \times (5 \times \mathbf{b} - (5 \times E(\mathbf{b}))) \\
&= E(5 \times (\mathbf{b} - E(\mathbf{b})) \times 5 \times (\mathbf{b} - E(\mathbf{b}))) \\
&= E(25 \times (\mathbf{b} - E(\mathbf{b})) \times (\mathbf{b} - E(\mathbf{b})) \\
&= 25 \times E((\mathbf{b} - E(\mathbf{b})) \times (\mathbf{b} - E(\mathbf{b}))) = 25 \times V(\mathbf{b}).
\end{aligned}
$$

In general, $V(x \times \mathbf{f}) = x \times x \times V(\mathbf{f})$ for any random variable $\mathbf{f}$ and number x. When you multiply a random variable by a number, you multiply its variance by the square of that number.

Variance of the sum, f + g

$$
\begin{aligned}
V(\mathbf{f} + \mathbf{g}) &= E((\mathbf{f} + \mathbf{g} - E(\mathbf{f} + \mathbf{g})) \times (\mathbf{f} + \mathbf{g} - E(\mathbf{f} + \mathbf{g}))) \\
(\text{E is linear}) &= E(((\mathbf{f} - E(\mathbf{f})) + (\mathbf{g} - E(\mathbf{g}))) \times (\mathbf{f} - E(\mathbf{f})) + (\mathbf{g} - E(\mathbf{g})))) \\
(\text{multiply out}) &= E((\mathbf{f} - E(\mathbf{f}) \times (\mathbf{f} - E(\mathbf{f})) + E((\mathbf{f} - E(\mathbf{f}) \times (\mathbf{g} - E(\mathbf{g})) \\
&\quad + E((\mathit{f} - E(\mathbf{f}) \times (\mathbf{g} - E(\mathbf{g})) + E((\mathbf{g} - E(\mathbf{g}) \times (\mathbf{g} - E(\mathbf{g})) \\
(\text{recognize V}) &= V(\mathbf{f}) + 2 \times E((\mathbf{f} - E(\mathbf{f}) \times (\mathbf{g} - E(\mathbf{g}))) + V(\mathbf{g}).
\end{aligned}
$$

The variance of the sum fails to be the sum of the variances because of an extra term, $E((\mathbf{f} - E(\mathbf{f}) \times (\mathbf{g} - E(\mathbf{g}))$. This extra term is called the Covariance of $\mathbf{f}$ and $\mathbf{g}$, written $CoV(\mathbf{f},\mathbf{g})$. It is a measure of the extent to which sampled values of $\mathbf{f}$ and $\mathbf{g}$ tend to go up or down together. If they do not tend at all to go up or down together, i.e., if they tend to assume their sampled values independently, $CoV(\mathbf{f},\mathbf{g})$ is 0, and we say that $\mathbf{f}$ and $\mathbf{g}$ are independent random variables.

In general, $V(\mathbf{f} + \mathbf{g}) = V(\mathbf{f}) + V(\mathbf{g}) + 2 \times CoV(\mathbf{f},\mathbf{g})$. Thus it is clear that the variance of the sum is the sum of the variances, only in the case that $\mathbf{f}$ and $\mathbf{g}$ are independent random variables. Covariance is an interesting concept to which we will return in Chapter 7.

All these concepts and generalizations associated with expected values and variances apply equally to random variables with continuous distributions, by replacing discrete sums with calculus integrals. For example, consider again $\mathbf{u}$, a random variable uniformly distributed over [0.0, 1.0]. Because the expected value of a random variable (or equivalently of its distribution) is an indication of the probabilistic middle of its range of values, you might guess that $E(\mathbf{u}) = 0.5$, which is correct, as you have seen earlier in this section. The probability density function for $\mathbf{u}$ is the function that assigns the value 1 to every x in the interval [0.0, 1.0]. Thus, by integral calculus, $E(\mathbf{u})$ is the definite integral between 0.0 and 1.0 of the function $1 \times x$ taken with respect to x. As you have seen, this is the area under the triangle bounded above by the line from (0,0) to (1,1), which is 0.5. The expected value of $\mathbf{b}$ with $p = 0.5$ is $E(\mathbf{b}) = 0.5$, the same as $E(\mathbf{u})$. For $\mathbf{b}$ with

$p = 0.5$, $V(\mathbf{b})$ is $0.5 \times 0.5 = 0.25$. You might guess that $V(\mathbf{u}) = V(\mathbf{b})$, but in fact, $V(\mathbf{u})$ is considerably less than $V(\mathbf{b})$, because many possible sample values of $\mathbf{u}$ can be very close to its mean.

The variance of $\mathbf{u}$

To calculate the variance of $\mathbf{u}$ with calculus, you would need to evaluate the definite integral of

$$1 \times (x - 0.5) \times (x - 0.5)$$

between 0.0 and 1.0 with respect to x. If you can do basic integral calculus, you can confirm that

$$V(\mathbf{u}) = 1/3 - 1/2 + 1/4 = 1/12$$

which is much less than 1/4. The integral calculus in this example is accessible to first-year calculus students, but in general, the integral calculus expressions that arise from doing arithmetic with continuous probability distributions can be very complex. Sometimes even trained mathematicians cannot manipulate some of those expressions with calculus to get answers. However, as you become more familiar with the basic concepts of doing arithmetic with random variables by practicing with simple, discrete (i.e., not continuous) examples, you will be able to manipulate continuous distributions computationally, without any need for integral calculus. For example, to estimate $E(\mathbf{u})$ computationally, you could write an EXCEL macro with these instructions:

```
EV = 0.0 'Initialize expected value at 0.0
For I = 1 To 10000
   EV = EV + Rnd 'Add up 10000 samples of u
   Next I
EV = EV / 10000 'Divide the sum by the number of samples
```

To estimate V(**u**) you could use instructions like those above:

```
VAR = 0.0
For I = 1 To 10000
    X = Rnd 'You cannot use Rnd in place of X below. Why?
    VAR = VAR + (X - 0.5) * (X - 0.5)
    Next I
VAR = VAR / 10000
```

Of course, your macros would still have to name and type EV, VAR, X, and I, initialize the random number generator, and write the estimates, EV and VAR, on a spreadsheet. I ran my macro to estimate variance three times and got the estimates 0.0820, 0.0836, and 0.0835. The theoretical value of V(**u**) is 1/12 (0.0833 …) but for statistical argument, close estimates are usually adequate. Actually, because of questionable assumptions and asymptotic approximations, many of the values produced by classical statistics are just estimates anyway, and sometimes not even very good ones.

You can use the linear operator property of Expected Value for any random variables, and of Variance for independent random variables, to determine theoretically the value of many expressions, such as $E(\mathbf{u} + \mathbf{u} + \mathbf{u}) = 1.5$ and $V(\mathbf{u} + \mathbf{u} + \mathbf{u}) = 3/12 = 1/4$. For these and/or similar expressions, you can practice by determining their values theoretically, and then writing macros to estimate them.

5 | More programming and statistical concepts

5.1   Re-sampling data

A question

I went fly fishing with my friend John. We caught 14 fish. He was casting a Blue Bobber and caught six fish, and I was casting a Grimacing Willy and caught eight fish. I wondered, "Do Blue Bobbers tend to catch the same size fish as Grimacing Willies?"

To answer this question using the methods I have presented, I need to: (1) use as data the 14 fish we caught, measured by weight and structured into two groups based on which fly caught them; (2) use as a test statistic a number, calculated from the data, that sums up how much heavier are the fish caught on Blue Bobbers than the fish caught on Grimacing Willies; (3) hypothesize a specific probability mechanism that represents the hypothesis that weights of fish caught on Blue Bobbers are not different from weights of fish caught on Grimacing Willies; (4) put that mechanism in motion to compute a large number of data sets, each similar in structure to the one observed, but constituting a sample of the hypothesis; (5) from each data set calculate a value of the test statistic; (6) sort these values and report them as an estimate of the probability distribution predicted by the hypothesis that fish weights are not different; (7) see where in this predicted distribution the observed weight difference falls; and finally (8) decide whether the observed data seem to be consistent with the hypothesis.

With this example, I will show you some concepts and techniques useful for implementing some of these basic steps. In this case, the structure of the data is pretty straightforward, as is the nature of the question I want to ask. But I will not have finished assembling the basic ingredients until I have invented a test statistic and hypothesized a random-data-generating mechanism.

Choose a test statistic

Recall that a test statistic is any number that I can calculate from data to use as a summary of those data for the purpose of testing a hypothesis. As you have seen, it is important to choose a test statistic that accurately reflects the concept in question. In classical statistics, you are often required to calculate the statistic in a very specific, often somewhat complicated, way. This is because the random-data-generating mechanism and test statistic have already been determined to ensure that the predicted probability distribution is one that has already been calculated. Limiting the hypotheses and test statistics in this way limits the questions you can ask and test. Also, when these choices have already been made for you, it is tempting not to bother to learn exactly what hypotheses and test statistics are driving your statistical results, especially because it is often quite difficult; this failure makes you a less responsible scientist.

To help answer the question about dry flies, I could choose as a test statistic the average weight of the six fish caught on the Blue Bobber minus the average weight of the eight fish caught on the Grimacing Willy. I would predict that its value would be near zero if I had hypothesized that the two lures caught the same size fish. This seems like a straightforward and reasonable test statistic that well represents the question. But it is worth thinking about it more, now that you are free (and responsible) for structuring your own test statistic to really ask what you want. Actually, I did not mind catching a varying number of little fish while trying to catch a few big ones. For my interests, a better test statistic might be the sum of the weights of the three heaviest fish caught on the Blue Bobber minus the sum of the three heaviest fish caught on the Grimacing Willy. This leaves out all those pesky little fish that happened to get caught along the way. If this statistic better reflects what you are asking or arguing about, then it would be a better one for you to use in your argument. In any case, you are free to decide what makes most sense to you for your purpose, because your computational approach does not require that your hypothesis predict a pre-calculated distribution for your test statistic. You will calculate your own predicted distribution.

Design the macro

I wrote a program to predict a probability distribution for a test statistic that will enable me to answer the question, Do the two dry flies catch the same size three biggest fish? I started as usual by giving names and designating types to some places in the computer's memory to structure and hold a data set. When I wrote this macro, I called it FISH, and started it like this:

```
Sub FISH()
Dim WEIGHTBB(10), WEIGHTGW(10) As Single
Dim NCWBB, NCWGW As Integer
Dim I As Integer
```

Place I contains which fish (We each named our fish 1, 2, ... in the order we caught them); NCWBB contains the number caught with a Blue Bobber and NCWGW contains the number caught with a Grimacing Willy. WEIGHTBB(I) contains in place, I, the weight of the fish caught on a Blue Bobber and WEIGHTGW(I) contains in place, I, the weight of the fish caught on a Grimacing Willy. These places contain the observed data set, structured in a way that preserves the distinctions related to the question.

Next, I needed to decide where on a spreadsheet to enter the data so that my macro could read them. Anywhere convenient would be fine, so long as my macro reads them from the right place. So I decided to put the Blue Bobber data in column 1 and the Grimacing Willy data in column 2, with row 1 containing the number of fish caught with each fly and the remaining rows containing the fish weights.

Thus my macro reads data from the spreadsheet like this:

```
NCWBB = Worksheets("Sheet1").Cells(1,1)
For I = 1 To NCWBB
    WEIGHTBB(I) = Worksheets("Sheet1").Cells(I+1,1)
    Next I
NCWGW = Worksheets("Sheet1").Cells(1,2)
For I = 1 To NCWGW
    WEIGHTGW(I) = Worksheets("Sheet1").Cells(I+1,2)
    Next I
```

Now that I have places for data, I can use them to calculate a value for my test statistic. In my macro, this calculation came next, but I will leave the description of these details for later.

Not different mean same random process

The hypothesis in question states that the weights of the fish caught on the two flies are not different, except possibly for little fish that are not interesting. If the value of the test statistic turns out to be surprisingly too high or too low (depending on how it is defined) when compared with the probability distribution predicted for it by the hypothesis, then I could argue that one lure is better at catching big fish than the other. Next I needed to describe a random-data-generating mechanism to make that hypothesis computationally specific. Because the hypothesis states that the weights of big fish caught on either fly are not different, an effective approach is to use the same random-data-generating mechanism to produce the weights of fish caught with either type of dry fly. With this approach, The fish weights are not different, means that they are produced by the same random-data-generating mechanism. Of course, I still have to choose that mechanism.

I would like that mechanism to reflect the natural variation among fish weights, while minimizing any extraneous or irrelevant variation. Obviously, I do not intend for the concept, the same size, to mean exactly the same size, but more like, the same sort of sizes. It is effective to sample a random variable to implement this intent. Thus, I will independently sample the SAME fish-weight random variable to simulate the size of the next fish caught, whether that fish is caught on a Blue Bobber or on a Grimacing Willy.

Re-sampling data

To make my argument plausible, I still have to invent a fish-weight random variable that comes up with weights that are representative of the fish being caught. To be credible, any possible weights that this random variable might assume must include at least the weights that were actually observed. One approach would be to hypothesize that ANY size within the observed range, and perhaps a few just outside, might be possible; if I could hypothesize plausible probabilities for these possibilities, I would have a random variable that I could sample to generate fish weights. This approach has been common in classical statistics, and I will discuss it in more detail later. However, only for the weights actually observed do I have hard evidence for their possibility or frequency. So another approach is to hypothesize a fish-weight random variable that assigns one of the observed sizes, with a probability proportional to its observed frequency.

The approach described above is called re-sampling data. To sample a random variable defined by re-sampling data I combined all the observed fish weights into a single array, which I named POOL, with TNOF (total number of fish) weights in it. After my macro read the data from "Sheet1", I wrote these instructions to load POOL().

```
TNOF = 0
For I = 1 To NCWBB
    TNOF = TNOF + 1
    POOL(TNOF) = WEIGHTBB(I)
    Next I
For I = 1 To NCWGW
    TNOF = TNOF + 1
    POOL(TNOF) = WEIGHTGW(I)
    Next I
```

Instructions to sample this fish weight random variable.

```
I = 0
Do Until I = NCWBB
  I = I + 1
  X = Rnd * TNOF
  J = 1
  Do Until J >= X
     J = J + 1
     Loop ' J >= X
  WEIGHTBB(I) = POOL(J)
  Loop ' I =
I = 0
Do Until I = NCWGW
  I = I + 1
  X = Rnd * TNOF
  J = 1
  Do Until J >= X
     J = J + 1
     Loop ' J >= X
  WEIGHTGW(I) = POOL(J)
  Loop ' I =
```

Based on re-sampling data to create a simulated data set, I used "Rnd" to choose fish weights equiprobably from the pool of observed weights, like this.

I use the function "Rnd" to put a value of type "Single" in place X; then to create the appropriate index for POOL my macro has to find the smallest integer J that is still greater than X. I use this fish-weight random variable to simulate data sets with the same structure as the data set we observed, assigning plausible values to the weights of the fish caught on each of the two dry flies, but under the hypothesis that the same mechanism is operating to assign weights to fish caught with either fly.

Overview

After reading the data, my macro calculates the sums of the weights of the three heaviest fish caught on each fly, subtracts this sum for Grimacing Willy from this sum for Blue Bobber and puts this signed difference in DIF. This signed difference is the value of my test statistic calculated from the observed data. The sign is important because, if I reject the hypothesis, the sign will tell me which fly is catching bigger fish. After my macro has simulated a data set, it calculates SIMDIF in exactly the same way that it calculated DIF, except it used the simulated data set instead of the observed data. SIMDIF holds a sample of the random variable that my test statistic became when I hypothesized that our data were generated by a random process. This random variable has the probability distribution predicted by my hypothesis. My macro writes this sample (SIMDIF) to a column of a spreadsheet, and compares it with the observed value (DIF) to increment the significance counters, SIGHI and SIGLO. To estimate the predicted probability distribution, this process is repeated 1000 (or more) times. To calculate DIF and to compare 1000 samples of the probability distribution predicted by the hypothesis for DIF, I wrote these instructions.

```
' Instructions to calculate the observed value of DIF
Worksheets("Sheet1").Cells(1,3) = DIF
SIGHI = 0
SIGLO = 0
Randomize
For NS = 1 To 1000
```

```
    *** Instructions like those above to re-sample data to
simulate a random data set
    *** Instructions to calculate the value of SIMDIF
for this simulated data set, i.e., exactly the same
instructions used to calculate the value for DIF from
observed data
    Worksheets("Sheet1").Cells(NS,4) = SIMDIF
    If SIMDIF >= DIF Then SIGHI = SIGHI + 1
    If SIMDIF <= DIF Then SIGLO = SHGLO + 1
    Next NS
Worksheets("Sheet1").Cells(1,5) = SIGHI
Worksheets("Sheet1").Cells(2,5) = SIGLO
```

This way of re-sampling data to simulate a data set overwrites our observed data set. So, my macro must use our observed data to calculate an observed value of the test statistic before it overwrites the space with simulated data. Of course, at the beginning of my macro, I will need to name and type the places in which to put the observed and simulated values of the test statistic, to count up the realized significances, and to count simulations.

Style

The EXCEL macro interpreter treats more than one blank space the same as a single space. In the macro editor, before and after reserved single character symbols, such as =, (, <, etc., no space is required, but may be inserted for style. Names that you have given to places in memory are shown in capitals in this book and must have at least one space, or one of the reserved single character symbols, to delimit them in the macro editor. Most other compilers or interpreters use the same or similar conventions to enable you to write your source statements in a style that will let you read them more easily to see whether you have accurately implemented your intent. Style happens when you insert new lines and blanks (indentation), how and where you make comments (after a prime mark,'), how you choose to name places in memory, what you capitalize, etc. If you do not already have a personal programming style, you are urged to adopt the style used in this book until you have enough experience to develop your own personal style. In any case, use consistently some style that makes sense to you. Style is important to help you read your macro statements to ensure accuracy and to more efficiently find and correct mistakes. Every good programmer makes mistakes when creating programs; every good programmer adheres carefully to a personal style to help find and correct mistakes, to facilitate changes, and to make it easier to reuse blocks of statements in new programs.

Efron

Re-sampling data to create a random variable to represent the natural variation underlying some phenomena of interest seemed overly simplistic to many. Many of the possible values for the real random variable that produced the observed values may not have been represented. Re-sampling data might not be variable enough to represent the full scope of natural variation adequately. Efron (1979) tested this question. His approach was to sample a well-known distribution, such as the normal distribution, which we will discuss in Section 6.3, a number of times. He then re-sampled this pool of samples to estimate parameters of interest. The same parameters were also estimated using established techniques of mathematical statistics. The two estimates were compared, and even for moderate numbers of initial samples, they were similar. Efron's remarkable result shook up the statistical world and launched the rapid growth of data re-sampling methods, sometimes called boot-strap methods, for reasons that escape me. Techniques of computational statistics based on re-sampling data can be especially effective when underlying distributions are not known, or where effective mathematical techniques to manipulate distributions have not yet been invented. In fact, Efron and Tibshirani (1986) have shown how computational statistics can be used to determine the accuracy of estimations made by classical (mathematical) statistics. Many of you will not be able to read these publications meaningfully because they are technical, but I give you their citations so you can be aware of them.

Fossil teeth – The example above uses a test statistic based on only the three biggest fish caught by each fly; it illustrates the power and flexibility of computational approaches to statistical argument, because this test statistic would challenge even the most competent mathematical statistician to predict its probability distribution.

This example may seem a little far-fetched. However, Virginia is interested in the following question. Scientists discovered a cave in China that seems to have been occupied by people between about 800 000 years before present and about 500 000 years before present. During the excavation of the cave, the only human remains recovered were about 50 molar teeth, although much other archaeological evidence of human occupancy was recovered. When homologous (from the same place in the jaw) molars were compared, the average size of the teeth from the earlier (lower) part of the cave was larger than the average size of the teeth from the later (upper) part of the cave. One group of anthropologists argued that either evolutionary trends over this time period selected for smaller teeth in these people, or these people were replaced in this location by people with smaller teeth. Another group of anthropologists argued that there was no change in tooth size comparing the earlier and later groups of people who occupied this cave during this time span, but there was a change in their social practices that resulted in men indulging in more dangerous activities far from the cave (war or hunting), which was more likely to kill them there, while women remained in the vicinity of the cave performing more domestic activities and thus were more likely to die in the cave. Because female people have had on average slightly smaller teeth than male people, even before 800 000 years ago, this change in social structure would account for a decrease in average size of teeth recovered from the later group. Clearly, difference in average tooth sizes of teeth from upper vs lower cave is not a statistic that she can use to distinguish these two explanations.

In either case, the biggest teeth in either group would be more likely to be male. If the size of a male tooth sampled the same random variable for both the earlier and later groups (social explanation), then the difference of the average sizes of the biggest few teeth in each group would be near zero or only slightly larger for the earlier group (because it contains more males), and this observed difference should be near the middle of the probability distribution predicted by this hypothesis for this statistic. If evolution or replacement had resulted in a general reduction in maximum tooth size for males of the later group, the observed value of this statistic would be near a tail of this predicted distribution. A similar analysis could be done for females by looking at the smallest few teeth in each group.

You can see how the basic idea of the test statistic for the heaviest three fish applies to teeth in this case. Under the hypothesis that teeth size did not change over time (the social-change hypothesis) the predicted distribution for a biggest-three or littlest-three test statistic should have an expected value near zero. If the observed difference of the largest (male) or smallest (female) few teeth is near the middle of this predicted distribution, she could argue that the social-change hypothesis is more credible, but if the later biggest (smallest) few teeth were substantially smaller than the earlier few teeth, then she could argue that change of tooth size by evolution or replacement is more credible.

As usual, these estimates will have errors as a consequence of simulation, but these errors can be made (probably) smaller by simulating more data sets. However, these particular estimates may have errors as a consequence of the fact that she is simulating the social-change hypothesis, but she does not know exactly how many of the teeth in each group belong to males and how many belong to females, but presumably more in the earlier group than in the later group belong to males. Thus the expected value of her estimated predicted distribution should indicate that the average size of the largest (smallest) few teeth from the earlier group is slightly larger. With smaller amounts of data, or smaller amounts of change, it becomes more difficult to reject any hypothesis she simulates; in cases like these, competing hypotheses have to remain ambiguous. However, a competent statistical analysis whose answer is a definite maybe, will legitimize both hypotheses as possibly credible, which can help us to stop shouting at each other and get back to doing good science.

5.2   Procedures

Why write procedures?

To complete my macro to calculate a predicted probability distribution for a test statistic to see if I can argue that one fly caught bigger fish than the other, I still need to write the statements that calculate a value for that test statistic. I will want to use those statements in two places: once to calculate an observed value using the observed data, and then to calculate simulated values using simulated data. In such cases, it is often convenient to compose those statements in a procedure, also called a sub-routine, or a method, or a function, which you can call from different places in your macro to execute exactly the same statements over again using different data.

How to write a procedure

A procedure is just like a macro. In fact, macros ARE procedures called by EXCEL. The reserved word "Sub" that begins a macro is short for subroutine, which is what procedures were called by BASIC, the ancient programming language now used to program macros in EXCEL. I will use the word procedure to refer to a "Sub" that is called by another "Sub". To write a procedure, first you must give it a name. I named my procedure to calculate the difference between the three biggest fish, DIFBIG3(). It uses the arrays WEIGHTBB() and WEIGHTGW() and the numbers in NCWBB and NCWGW, to calculate the difference: the sum of the three biggest fish in array WEIGHTBB minus the sum of the three biggest fish in array WEIGHTGW. I want DIFBIG3 to put this difference in DIF when it calculates with observed data, but in SDIF when it calculates with simulated data. To do this, when I name BIGDIF3(), I name and type place DB3 inside the () like this: Sub DIFBIG3(DB3 As Single). To calculate DIF for observed data macro FISH uses the statement, BIGDIF3(DIF) but to calculate SDIF for simulated data it uses the statement, BIGDIF3(SDIF). On subsequent lines, I write instructions that compute a value for the test statistic, DB3, whose value will be placed in DIF or SDIF when BIGDIF3 executes. These instructions end with "EndSub", and are followed by macro, FISH, which reads data, simulates data, and reports results, as shown below:

```
Sub DIFBIG3 (DB3 As Single)
*** calculate a value for the test statistic in BD3
End Sub 'DIFBIG3
Sub FISH ()
*** read data from the spreadsheet (Cols 1&2)
Call DIFBIG3 (DIF)
Worksheets ("Sheet1") .Cells (1,3) = DIF
*** initialize significance counters
FOR NS = 1 To 1000
   *** Instructions to simulate a data set
   Call BIGDIF3 (SDIF)
   *** Instructions to increment significance counters
   Next NS
*** Instructions to report results (Col 4)
End Sub 'FISH
```

When FISH calls DIFBIG3(DIF), DIF plays the role of DB3 and the answer, i.e., the value of the test statistic calculated with the observed data, ends up in DIF. When FISH calls DIFBIG3(SDIF), SDIF plays the role of DB3 and a value of the test statistic calculated with simulated data ends up in SDIF. In this way, I compose the instructions once, but can ask them to be executed more than once in different places in my macro, putting the results of the calculations in different places.

Access to places

Places named and typed in a macro or procedure belong to that macro or procedure and are not usually available to other procedures. Because such places are named and used privately, other procedures can use the same names, but they refer to different places in the computer's memory. When macros or procedures call a procedure, some of their places can be made available to the procedure called by passing them in parentheses at the time of the call. DIF and SDIF are examples of places that belong to FISH, but that are made available to DIFBIG3 by passing them when BIGDIF3 is called.

DIFBIG3 also needs to use the data in WEIGHTBB and WEIGHTGW. Because these places will have the same name every time DIFBIG3 is called, an easier way to make them available to DIFBIG3 is to declare them at the module level, instead of inside macro FISH. This makes them available to any procedures in that module, in particular to the procedures and to the macro that calls them. To name and type places at the module level, do so outside macro FISH, before any statements that describe procedures or the macro that calls them. It is important NOT to name and type them again inside macro FISH or any of the procedures that it calls, because this makes local again places with those names. This is the beginning of my module:

```
Dim WEIGHTBB(10) As Single
Dim WEIGHTBB(10) As Single
Dim NCWBB As Integer
Dim NCWGW As Integer
```

Sub SORT

DIFBIG3 calculates a value for the test statistic by first sorting the tables WEIGHTBB and WEIGHTGW from heaviest to lightest. Then it adds into

DB3BB the weights of the first three fish in WEIGHTBB and it adds into DB3GW the weights of the first three fish in WEIGHTGW. Then it puts their difference in DIF or SDIF, whichever plays the role of DB3; Call DIFBIG3(DIF) makes DIF play the role of DB3 and Call DIFBIG3(SDIF) makes SDIF play the role of DB3. To sort, DIFFBIG3 calls procedure "SORT(L,TABLE())", which implements the so-called shell sort, devised by computer scientists to realize the maximum efficiency for general sort procedures. I wrote Sub SORT shown below to implement this algorithm:

```
Sub SORT(L as Integer, TABLE() As Single)
Dim HOLD As Single 'helps swap values
Dim I, J, M, N, JUMP As Integer
'indices, length of swap intervals
Dim DONE As Byte '1 will mean TRUE 0 will mean FALSE
JUMP = L
Do Until JUMP = 1 'Keep Looping until jump interval is only 1
   J = 1
   Do Until J * 2 >= JUMP 'Find least Integer >= JUMP/2
     J = J + 1
     Loop 'J * 2
   JUMP = J
   DONE = 0
   Do Until DONE = 1
'Compare all values in intervals of length JUMP
     DONE = 1
     M = 0
     Do Until M >= (L - JUMP)
       M = M + 1
       N = M + JUMP
       If TABLE(M) < TABLE(N) Then 'Switch larger value up
         HOLD = TABLE(M)
         TABLE(M) = TABLE(N)
         TABLE(N) = HOLD
         DONE = 0
         End If 'TABLE( Done switching
       Loop 'M >= Done comparing values in this interval
     Loop 'DONE Done comparing all intervals of length JUMP
   Loop 'JUMP Done comparing all decreasing interval lengths
End Sub
```

The sub-routine SORT(L,TABLE()) sorts an array TABLE() with L values typed as Single so that its largest value is in place 1 and its smallest value is in place L. When you call SORT(L,TABLE()) in your macro, you substitute for L the number of places in the table you want to sort and you substitute for TABLE() the name of the table (with values of type Single) you want to sort. Put the statements defining "SORT(L,TABLE())" right after naming and typing module level places. Follow them with statements defining procedure, DIFBIG3.

BIGDIF3

My procedure DIFBIG3 looks like this:

```
Sub DIFBIG3 (DB3 As Single)
    ' External: WEIGHTBB(), NCWBB, WEIGHTGW(), NCWGW
Dim I As Integer
Dim S3BB, S3GW As Single
Call (SORT(NCWBB, WEIGHTBB())
S3BB = 0
For I = 1 TO 3
    S3BB = S3BB + WEIGHTBB(I)
    Next I
Call (SORT(NCWGW, WEIGHTGW())
S3GW = 0
For I = 1 To 3
    S3GW = S3GW + WEIGHTGW(I)
    DB3 = S3BB - S3GW
End Sub 'DIFBIG3
```

After all of this come the statements that define macro FISH() itself. While writing these statements, I saved my workbook at frequent intervals; I called it FISH.XLS to remind myself what macro it contains. Special procedures like BIGDIF3(DB3) are useful because you can call them more than once to do the same job in different places in the same macro. More general procedures, such as "SORT(L,TABLE())", are useful not only because you can call them more than once in a macro to do the same job again in a different place, but also because you can copy them into other macros to do the same job in different contexts. You may want to insert a new module, name it SORT, and copy the SORT procedure into it, so you can find it again easily.

5.3   Testing procedures

Except for the smallest tasks, I have never written a program that ran correctly the first time. You should not expect the macros that you write to run correctly the first time either. Good programmers realize that not just designing and composing, but also testing and correcting, are part of the process. In fact, many good programmers design tests (and test data) as part of the design phase of programming. Thus, they specify in advance what they will accept as evidence that a procedure is running correctly. It is virtually impossible to ensure that your program (or anyone else's) will not make mistakes when run with new data; a program can be guaranteed to make no more mistakes only if it is never run again. In spite of this cynical stance, there are steps you can take to make your macros and procedures more reliable.

Testing SORT

Some have been thoroughly tested. In the case of procedures such as "SORT(L,TABLE())" that will be useful in other macros, I suggest that you maintain them in separate modules. To do this, create a new module in your EXCEL macro editor and name it SORT. Copy the statements above that define "SORT(L,TABLE())" and follow them with a macro called CALLSORT(), which loads a small table with values of type "Single", writes these values on "Sheet1" (somewhere), calls "SORT(L,TABLE())", and writes the sorted values on "Sheet1" (somewhere else). If the table is sorted, this will help you be more confident that your "SORT(L,TABLE())" procedure is running correctly. In the macro below, I named and typed an array called ALIST() with 10 places; then I loaded it with 10 random numbers between 0.0 and 1.0 using the function "Rnd"; then I wrote the table on a spreadsheet; then I called "SORT(10,ALIST())"; and finally I wrote the sorted table on the same spreadsheet. So now you try it. After you have challenged yourself to your satisfaction, look below at how I did it. Notice that I speak of what my macro is doing as if I were doing it. Once the concepts are clear, it is easier to say how to do things in this way.

```
Sub CALLSORT()
Dim ALIST(10) As Single
Dim I As Integer
MsgBox("Begin CALLSORT")
Randomize
For I = 1 TO 10
    ALIST(I) = Rnd
    Worksheets("Sheet1").Cells(I,1) = ALIST(I)
    Next I
Call SORT(10,ALIST())
For I = 1 TO 10
    Worksheets("Sheet1").Cells(I,2) = ALIST(I)
    Next I
MsgBox("End CALLSORT")
End Sub 'CALLSORT
```

If the call to "SORT(10,ALIST())" produces a sorted table, then you have some reason to believe that Sub SORT(L, TABLE()) is working. If it is not already there, you can now cut and paste it near the top of your FISH macro (which should be in its own module), follow it with your sub-routine, DIFBIG3(DB3), and finally with your macro FISH. It is a good idea to test "SORT(L,TABLE())" to have some reason to believe that it is working the way you intend before using it in a larger context.

Test data

When you have written enough of your macro FISH() so that it writes DIF in column 3 of your spreadsheet, compile and run it to see if DIF has the value you expect. To do this, you will have to make up some data to enter in columns 1 and 2. Start with simple data for which you can easily calculate DIF yourself. For example, in column 1, enter fish weights that are all 1.0 except for three fish that weigh 3.0, and in column 2, fish weights that are all 2.0 except for three that are 4.0. Now DIF should be $9.0 - 12.0 = -3.0$.

When DIFBIG3(DIF) seems to be getting the right answer, write the rest of your macro, but simulate only once (not 1000 times). After a data structure has been simulated, write the values for WEIGHTBB() and WEIGHTGW() in columns 5 and 6 of your spreadsheet and the value for

SDIF in column 7. Do the simulated values look like they have been re-sampled from POOL()? If not, then look carefully at your statements; compare them with the examples above. Write the values on your spreadsheet; sometimes the wrong values can suggest what is wrong. If the simulated values look plausible, then use them to calculate on paper the value of SDIF. Is this the same value reported by your macro? If so, then you have some reason to believe that your macro is calculating SDIF correctly.

When things look OK, run your macro to simulate 100 data sets and write them in a column of your spreadsheet. When your macro has finished, ask EXCEL to sort that column. Take a look; are those values of SDIF plausible? EXCEL can easily handle a column of up to 1000 simulated values, so it is usually a good idea to write up to that many in a column to check that the values are all plausible, even if you are using significance counters like SIGHI and SIGLO. Also you may be interested to see the shape of the predicted distribution estimated by a sorted column of simulated values.

Infinite loop

One of the most mystifying kinds of mistakes you can make is one that results in your macro running forever; it never stops. When testing macros the way I am describing here, they should always finish instantly. If they are still running after a few seconds, there is almost certainly something wrong. Usually if you press the escape (Esc) or the Pause or the Break key, this will interrupt the running of your macro. Sometimes you may need to hold down the control (Ctrl) key while pressing one of these keys. What works seems to vary with operating system or program context. Experiment to see what works for you. After you interrupt your program, return to the macro editor, bring down the run menu and click "Reset".

To experience a situation in which your program never stops, edit your SORT procedure to introduce this glitch; change the statement:

```
Do Until J * 2 >= JUMP
```

to the statement;

```
Do Until J * 2 > JUMP
```

Omitting the = is a mistake anyone could easily make. Now, edit your spreadsheet so that CALLSORT tries to sort a table with eight entries.

When J contains 2 and JUMP contains 4, the "Do Until" is supposed to stop, but in the glitched version it does not. If you have made this mistake correctly, when you run the macro to sort a table with eight entries, it will never stop. Try it now. See what keys (Esc, Ctrl Esc, etc.) interrupt your macro.

When you interrupt your macro, EXCEL puts you back in the macro editor. Pull down the "Run" menu and click "Reset". Then put the cursor in front of the statement JUMP = J. Next pull down the "Debug" menu and click on "Run to cursor". This runs your macro until the next statement that it would execute is the one following the cursor. This keeps your macro from running forever, but also allows you to see what is in places in the computer's memory at this point, using the Watch window, in the lower right. Pull down the Debug menu again and click, Add watch. A box will open asking you for the name of the place you would like to watch, i.e., whose contents you would like to see. Enter J. J and its contents should show up in the watch window. If you continue to "Run to cursor" you can see that J's contents are not what they should be. This will suggest that you check statements that alter the contents of J, looking again carefully at "Sub SORT", as shown above.

The watch window

In this exercise, you know what is the mistake because you made it on purpose to see what would happen. Of course, when you make mistakes by mistake, you will not know what they are, and finding them may be challenging. I cannot tell you mechanically how to find your mistakes. Finding mistakes is part of the art of being a good programmer. I can give some advice based on my own experience. A second pair of eyes can really help a lot. As I have suggested before, work in pairs, if possible. In my experience, the watch window is a two-edged sword; it is a powerful tool, but you can waste a lot of time using it mindlessly. The combination of "Run to cursor" and "Watch" is effective if your macro won't stop. Otherwise, I have found it more effective to write my macros in small steps, writing intermediate results on my spreadsheet at each step, until things look OK.

Testing PERMUTE

Another collection of statements that you might find useful to put into a procedure to reuse in your other macros are those that permute an array, such as appeared in the earlier examples, CARPEL() and PERIOD(). Look at PERIOD to find those statements. Then open your macro editor and insert a new module (call it PERMUTE), and copy those statements. After you copy them, modify them to become more general. As a model, use the name of procedure "Sub SORT(L, TABLE())" to name "PERMUTE(L As Byte, TABLE(100) As Byte)". Now you could use this sub-routine in macro PERIOD with the statement, "Call PERMUTE(42,UOD())". When you define the procedure "Sub PERMUTE, TABLE()" should have type "Byte" because UOD() contains values of type "Byte". The places, NL, K, X, J, and HOLD are now private to Sub PERMUTE, so they must be named and typed at the beginning of the definition of Sub PERMUTE. Follow the statements for Sub PERMUTE with a small macro, name it CALLPERMUTE(), that reads a sequence of a few values from a spreadsheet, calls "PERMUTE(L, TABLE())" and writes a randomly chosen permutation of that sequence back to the spreadsheet. Use the macro, CALLSORT(), as a model. Run the macro CALLPERMUTE() to help ensure that procedure PERMUTE() is working OK before you cut and paste it into another context where you want to use it.

After you have challenged yourself to your satisfaction, look below to see how I did it:

```
Sub PERMUTE (L As Byte, TABLE (100) As byte)
Dim NL, K, J, HOLD As Byte
Dim X As Single
Randomize   'Initialize the random number generator, maybe
NL = L  'Number of unchosen places in TABLE() left to permute
For K = 1 To L-1  'Choose a random place to swap L - 1 times
    X = Rnd * NL  'generate a random number between 0.0 and 1.0
    J = 1  'then multiply by NL so that 0.0 <= X <= NL
    Do Until J > X  'Find the smallest Integer J larger than X
        J = J + 1
        Loop
    If J < NL Then
        HOLD = TABLE (J)   'Use J to index TABLE () and swap with
        TABLE (J) = TABLE (NL)   'last unchosen place
        TABLE (NL) = HOLD
        End If
    NL = NL - 1 'Decrement NL
    Next K
End Sub
```

```
Sub CALLPERMUTE()
Dim ALIST(10) As Byte
Dim R, C As Byte
MsgBox("Begin CALLPERMUTE")
For R = 1 To 10
    ALIST(R) = Worksheets("Sheet1").Cells(1,R)
    Next R
Call PERMUTE(10, ALIST())
For R = 1 To 10
    Worksheets("Sheet1").Cells(2,R) = ALIST(R)
    Next R
MsgBox("End CALLPERMUTE")
End Sub
```

For a little more practice correcting mistakes, imagine that you had forgotten to multiply Rnd by NL when loading X. To check this out, edit PERMUTE by putting a prime in front of * when loading X; the statement should look like: X = Rnd ' * NL ... Now X always has a number between 0.0 and 1.0, so that J always turns out to contain 1. This will result in a permutation of TABLE, but not a very random one. Imagine what permutation it would produce. Then run your CALLPERMUTE macro to see what permutation was produced. Unlike the SORT procedure, where there is only one way to correctly sort a table, when random processes are involved, there are typically many possibly correct answers. One example may not be very good evidence that a random procedure is working OK. So modify CALLPERMUTE so that it permutes several times by enclosing the Call PERMUTE, and the statements that write, in a For loop, like this:

```
For C = 1 To 10
    Call PERMUTE(10, ALIST())
    For R = 1 To 10
        Worksheets("Sheet1").Cells(C+2,R) = ALIST(R)
        Next R
    Next C
```

If you run this with PERMUTE, glitched as I suggested above, you will see a pattern of non-random permutations that will alert you to the possibility that something is wrong. This does not tell you how to find what it is, but it does help defend you from the worst kind of mistake, which is getting wrong answers without realizing it. Of course, in this case you know what the mistake is because you made it on purpose. But if you did not know, how could you find it? You could compare your statements to those in CARPEL or PERIOD. In general, if you were copying statements from another program, comparing them would be a good start. Otherwise, a technique I have found effective is to get out my paper and pencil and take the role of the computer myself. I usually do this first, before I resort to "Watch". In any case, finding and correcting mistakes is an important part of the art of programming; we all have to practice and be patient with it.

6 | Parametric distributions

6.1   Basic concepts

Parametric distributions are used extensively in classical statistics because mathematicians have manipulated their calculating formulas to devise test statistics whose predicted distributions are among the pre-calculated ones, some of which are listed in the backs of older statistics books. In addition, if a member of a parametric family adequately describes the variation in data of interest, these data can be used to estimate values for parameters; the name of the family together with values for its parameters make a useful summary description of that variation. Parametric distributions can also help define a hypothesized random process when you take a computational approach to statistical argument.

Binary distributions

Consider again a binary random variable **b** with possible values 1 and 0 and a distribution given by $\Pr(\mathbf{b} = 1) = \mathrm{p}$. Specified in this way, the random variable, **b**, is chosen from a large class of random variables that differ with respect to the mechanisms that sample them, but always have only two possible values, 0 and 1. Although the random variables in the class to which **b** belongs may differ, their distributions will be the same if $\Pr(\mathbf{b} = 1)$ is the same for both. We use the word, family, to refer to a collection of distributions that all have the same form, such as all the distributions for the random variable, **b**, but differ by the value of a number, such as p, which we call a parameter. Distributions that can be easily specified by designating the family to which they belong and specifying the value of a parameter (or sometimes the values of two or a few parameters), are called parametric distributions. Well-known families have names. The distribution of the random variable, **b**, belongs to a family named binary distributions.

Binomial distributions

These constitute another family of parametric distributions. A random variable of the form of **sn**, as discussed in Chapter 4, has a binomial distribution. The random variable **sn** is sampled by adding n independent samples of a random variable like **b** with a binary distribution. To specify a distribution for **sn** we must specify not only $p = \Pr(\mathbf{b} = 1)$ but also n, the number of times **b** is independently sampled to get the values that are summed to determine a value for **sn**. Thus, binomial distributions have two parameters, (n,p). With values for these parameters, we can use the formula given in Section 4.3 to calculate probabilities like this:

$$\Pr(\mathbf{sn} = i) = p^i \times q^{(n-1)} \times [n, i]$$

where as before, $[n,i]$ are the binomial coefficients.

Because a binomial distribution arises from a simple, repeated mechanism, it may be a plausible analogy to some natural phenomenon of interest, and thus provide a good way to specify a probability mechanism to include in your hypothesis. For example, suppose you have been walking in a patch of woods and you notice that some animals have dug burrows into the ground near the base of a few of the trees. You wonder if these burrowing animals prefer to burrow on the north side or the south side of a tree. So you start counting the number of trees with a burrow on the north side and the number with a burrow on the south side. You find seven trees with nearby burrows of which five have burrows on the north and only two have burrows on the south. You wonder if something might be causing burrows to be dug more often on the north. To see whether you have any strong evidence that something is causing burrows to be dug more often on the north, you could hypothesize that it really did not matter where a burrow was dug. One way to test this would be to see if your observations were consistent with the hypothesis that a burrow is equally likely to occur on either side of a tree. You could imagine that observing a tree with a burrow is a mechanism for sampling **b**, with distribution $\Pr(\mathbf{b} = 1) = 1/2$, by setting **b** = 1 if there is a burrow on the north and **b** = 0 if there is a burrow on the south. You could hypothesize that the trees represent independent samples of **b**. This establishes an analogy between your observations and a sample of **s7**. Through this analogy, you can use the binomial distribution with $n = 7$

and $p = 1/2$ to calculate the significance of a test statistic, which could be s7 itself.

$$Pr(s7 \geq 5) = Pr(s7 = 5) + Pr(s7 = 6) + Pr(s7 = 7) = 29/128$$

This shows a weak trend, but not convincing evidence to reject the hypothesis. You could observe more burrows to make a stronger argument.

Parametric distributions arise from specific processes

Similar to binomial distributions, members of other parametric distribution families also arise from specific processes that we can understand and recognize through analogies with natural phenomena. It may be appropriate to specify a member of a parametric family of probability distributions as part of your hypothesis. You can do this even when you intend to calculate a predicted probability distribution for a test statistic you have designed yourself. Your statistic would need to be constrained only by your scientific objectives and the circumstances in which your data were, or will be, observed.

A good way to recognize such appropriateness is to understand the specific processes that produce the variation described by a random variable with a probability distribution chosen from a particular parametric family. The rest of Chapter 6 presents several other examples of such processes and their associated parametric distributions.

6.2   Poisson distribution

A random variable with a Poisson distribution sometimes naturally describes the consequence of the independent occurrence of things in space or of events in time. The Poisson family of parametric distributions arises as limiting cases of sequences of members of the binomial family of parametric distributions. To see how this happens, I will start with an example of a random variable with a binomial distribution. Then we will define a sequence of random variables starting with this one, and see where it goes at its limit. During the argument, pay attention to the analogy between the random variables and the natural situation they describe.

Trees in a savanna

Suppose you observe 75 trees in a 25 ha savanna. Recall that 1 ha (hectare) is about 2 ff (football fields). There are, on average, three trees per ha. Consider a particular ha. Even though the average is three trees, there might be only two or five or none if the trees really were spread through the savanna at random. At random always means as if sampling a probability distribution, so to make clear what at random means, we need to specify a probability distribution. In this case I define at random like this. Divide one ha up into n small areas, so small that two trees could not occupy the same small area, but not so small that two trees could not each occupy adjacent areas. Hypothesize that a tree occupies any particular little area with probability p and independently of whether other little areas are occupied by a tree. The n small areas in a ha represent n samples of **b**, a random variable with a binary distribution. The number of trees in our ha are counted by **sn**, which has a binomial distribution with parameters (n,p). Use the symbol m to stand for E(**sn**), the expected number of trees in a ha. We know that $m = np$, so that $p = m/n$. The idea of our example is that one hectare has a very large number, n, of places where a tree could grow. For example, if trees had to be at least 3 meters apart then n would be about 1000. Savannas have their trees widely spaced, so m would be quite small compared to n, and $p = m/n$ would be a very small fraction. With this in mind, we will manipulate the calculating formula for Pr(K trees) in order to put it into a form that, under these conditions, will approximate a much simpler expression, with only one parameter.

The calculating formula for binomial distribution gives:

$$\text{Pr}(K \text{ trees}) = \frac{n \times (n-1) \times .. \times (n-(K-1))}{1 \times 2 \times .. \times K} \times (m/n)^K \times (1-(m/n))^{(n-K)}$$

Recognize the quotient on the left as the binomial coefficient $[n,K]$, the number of ways to choose K things from a collection of n things.

First multiply by n^K and divide by the product of K ns, which is multiplying by an elaborate name for 1, shown on the left below:

$$\frac{(n^K) \times n \times (n-1) \times .. \times (n-(K-1)) \times (m/n)^K \times (1-m/n)^{(n-K)}}{(n \times n \times .. \times n) \times 1 \times 2 \times .. \times K}$$

Now move (n^K) inside $(m/n)^K$ to get $(n \times m/n)^K$, which equals m^K.

Then move the K ns from denominator respectively under the K factors above them in the numerator. Recall $x^{(a-b)} = x^a \times x^{-b} = x^a / x^b$ and use this fact to put $(1 - (m/n))^{-K}$ into the denominator, to get:

$$\frac{\frac{n}{n} \times \frac{(n-1)}{n} \times .. \times \frac{(n - (K-1))}{n} \times m^K \times (1 - (m/n))^n}{1 \times 2 \times .. \times K \times (1 - (m/n))^K}$$

Recall the special circumstances in our savanna: K, the number of trees, is a small whole number from 0 to 5 or 6, rarely more; n, the number of places, is huge, a thousand or more; and p, the probability of finding a tree in any particular place, is tiny. Thus the first K factors in the numerator, and $(1 - (m/n)$ in the last factor of the denominator, are each nearly 1. The product of not very many (relative to n) numbers, each nearly 1, is nearly 1. If we replace those factors, each nearly equal to 1, with 1 we get an approximation:

$$\frac{m^K \times (1 + (-m/n))^n}{1 \times 2 \times .. \times K}$$

Now imagine a sequence of random variables with binomial distributions in which n doubles, but m, the expected number of trees, remains the same. Moving along this sequence, the factors nearly equal to 1 get closer and closer to 1, so that the approximation above gets closer and closer to Pr(K trees). We say that this sequence of random variables has as its limit a random variable whose distribution IS this approximation.

An approximation of e

You may have noticed a computational problem with this. We have to multiply $(1 - m/n)$ by itself n times, which gets to be a hassle, even for a computer, as n grows truly astronomical. Fortunately, mathematicians have discovered e, a number whose approximate value is 2.7182818285, with the remarkable property that $(1 - m/n)^n$ gets closer and closer to e^{-m} as n gets larger and larger. So under the circumstances of the trees in our savanna,

$$\Pr(K \text{ trees in a ha}) = \frac{m^K \times e^{-m}}{1 \times 2 \times .. \times K} \text{ approximately}$$

In the case where $K = 0$, the denominator is 1 and the exponential, m to the K, is 1.

A random variable that assumes a possible value *K* with probability given by this formula is said to have a Poisson distribution with mean *m*. Poisson distributions constitute a family of parametric distributions with one parameter, *m*. You can use a Poisson distribution to define or conveniently approximate what you mean by the concept, distributed at random in space, for random variables like **nt** != number of trees in a ha. Especially now that you see where Poisson distributions come from, you can better recognize when to hypothesize one as an analogy to a natural phenomenon of interest.

Birds at a feeder

A Poisson distribution may also be appropriate to make clear what you meant by the concept, at random in time, to define a random variable to test a hypothesis. For example, on the hour for every daylight hour during a day, you looked out your window at your bird feeder and counted how many birds you saw feeding there. These are your counts:

> 1 3 4 2 0 4 2 1 3 2 0 3 1 2.

You wonder if the birds were scared away at the two times when you saw no birds. You can recognize an analogy to a random variable with a Poisson distribution that you sample by observing the number of birds, under a hypothesis that nothing scared them away. The mean number of birds observed at any given time is *m* = 28 / 14 = 2. The approximate probability of observing no birds at any given hour is given by *K* = 0 in the calculating formula. The product, e × e is a little over 7.3, so the probability of observing no birds at any given hour is just less than 1/7. With 14 independent observations, you would expect to observe no birds about twice. Is this evidence that something scared away the birds on the two occasions when you saw none? (hint: No)

The secret parameter

In practice, in addition to *m*, Poisson distributions usually have another parameter as well, which is the size of the area in which you are counting trees, or its conceptual equivalent. For example, if you counted trees in an ff instead of an ha you might hypothesize a Poisson distribution with smaller *m*.

It is possible for the observed placement of trees (or etc.) to be consistent with the hypothesis that the associated tree counting random variable has a Poisson distribution at one scale (like ha), but inconsistent with that hypothesis at another scale (like ff).

In natural situations such as those discussed above, when numbers of spatial (or temporal) occurrences observed do not seem to be consistent with a hypothesis that these observations are analogous to sampling a Poisson distributed random variable, often it is because there are too many samples at or near the expected value. We might interpret this case as evidence that the occurrences are too even or regular in space (or time) to be independent of one another. For example, if trees in the savanna could establish easily anywhere but excluded one another competing for limited water if they were closer to each other than say 20m, then we would expect to find 12 to 14 trees in every ff. We might observe too few samples at or near the expected number, i.e., too many with lower or higher counts. Something might be frightening the birds, or birds may have hours in the day when they prefer to come to your bird feeder.

How to sample a Poisson distribution in a macro

You may use a Poisson distributed random variable as part of a hypothesis, and sample its distribution to simulate data to estimate the predicted probability distribution for your test statistic. One way to do it is to calculate a cumulative Poisson distribution, and put it in an array, call it PD. You use PD to sample a Poisson distributed random variable. First sample the unit interval's continuous uniform distribution with "Rnd", and then find the place PD(J) that holds the smallest number larger than that sample. The index of that place is a sample of the Poisson distributed RV. I wrote these macro statements to do this:

```
Dim PD (20) As Single 'to hold cumulative Poisson distribution
Dim M, X As Single ' M is expected value, X samples u[0.0,1.0]
Dim K As Integer 'the value of the sample of the Poisson RV

*** Statements preceding the need to sample the RV
```

```
M = 3 ' or whatever the expected value might be
PD(1) = 1/Exp(M); ' load Pr(K=0) = e to the minus M into PD(1)
For K = 1 TO 20 ' load PD(2) with Pr(K=1), PD(3) with Pr(K=2) etc
    PD(K+1) = PD(K) x M / K
    Next K
For K = 1 To 20 ' convert PD to cumulative distribution
    PD(K+1) = PD(K+1) + PD(K)
    Next K
```

The instructions above introduce a new function, "Exp(M)", which returns e (2.7182818285..) raised to the power (content of) M.

Here is how I use PD to load K with a random sample:

```
X = Rnd 'a sample of u[0.0, 1.0]
K = 0
Do Until X <= PD(K+1)
K = K + 1
Loop 'X <= PD...
```

K now holds an integer 0 or greater. The most likely values are near the expected value; increasingly larger values become less likely, with values in excess of three times the expected very rare, because for a Poisson distribution variance equals expected value.

Ancient anthropology with genetic markers

Graciela is working in a well-equipped biological anthropology lab. She scrapes mitochondrial DNA from bones of 18 humans who were buried (and presumably lived) at a site in Meso-America about 3000 years ago. She amplifies the DNA to look for a genetic marker, which is present in 6 and absent in 12 of these folks. The bones of 11 humans are recovered from another location at the same site. By the same techniques, the marker is shown to be present in the mitochondrial DNA of nine of these folks. Using the same dating technology, she estimates that these 11 humans lived about 2500 years ago, about 20 generations later.

She wonders if the difference in marker frequency might have been a result of the population at this site having been invaded by a group with a higher marker frequency during the 500 years between samples. To test the need for such an explanation for the difference in frequency, she hypothesized that the marker frequency drifted for 20 generations. Based on archaeological evidence, she reasoned that a population of about 25 households occupied the site during the 500 years of interest. This might represent about 36 reproductive-aged women, who would be replaced by their female progeny every generation. She hypothesized that the genetic marker was not linked to genes with any selective advantage or disadvantage, so that a daughter in the replacing generation is equally likely to have been born to any mother in the generation being replaced. Mitochondria are inherited maternally, so the daughter will have the marker if and only if her mother did. If the population is stable, the expected number of daughters replacing a mother is $m = 1$. Under these conditions, the number of daughters replacing a mother is a random variable with the $m = 1$ Poisson distribution. Start with the observed 36 women, 12 of whom would have the marker; recall that 1/3 of the women in the older sample had the marker.

Challenge yourself to write a macro that uses my statements above to sample the Poisson distribution to simulate 20 generations of daughters replacing mothers. The fraction of women with the marker in the final population is your test statistic. Its distribution is predicted by the hypothesis that there was no invasion (Poisson). Simulate 1000 or more final populations from the observed starting population to estimate that predicted distribution. The observed value in the final population is 9/11. Compare this value with the predicted distribution to make an argument.

Stable population

Another way to simulate daughters replacing mothers under this hypothesis does not explicitly sample a Poisson distribution, even though the number of daughters replacing a mother still turns out to be approximately (i.e., in the limit) Poisson distributed. This way keeps the population size exactly the same from one generation to the next by choosing a mother equiprobably among all mothers and then putting her daughter in the replacement generation. I do this independently for each daughter to simulate a replacement generation. Then I choose equiprobably 11 daughters from this final population to calculate a simulated value for the test statistic.

6.3   Normal distribution

Standardization

Consider again a random variable with a binomial distribution specified by parameters (n,p). As before, we will call it **sn**. From Section 4.4 you know that $E(\textbf{sn}) = n \times p$, the expected value of the sum of n random variables, each with an expected value of p, and you know that $V(\textbf{sn}) = n \times p \times (1 - p)$, the variance of the sum of n independent random variables each with a variance of $p \times (1 - p)$. Once the values for n and p have been designated, the distribution for **sn** is fixed, so that its expected value, $E(\textbf{sn})$, and its variance, $V(\textbf{sn})$, are just constant numbers that are properties of that distribution; they are not themselves random variables. These numbers can be used to transform **sn** arithmetically into a new random variable, **sn#**, like this.

$$\textbf{sn\#}\,! = (\textbf{sn} - E(\textbf{sn}))/\text{SQRT}(V(\textbf{sn})))$$
$$= (\textbf{sn} - n \times p)/\text{SQRT}(n^*p^*(1 - p))$$

The random variable **sn#** has an expected value of 0 and a variance of 1. It is similar to **sn**, but its values have been centered around zero, and re-scaled to have a variance of 1. They were centered by subtracting the expected value, and rescaled by then dividing by the square root of the variance, which is called the standard deviation. Such centering and rescaling is called standardization.

   Although here a binomially distributed random variable was standardized, any random variable (with numerical values) can be standardized in the same way, by first subtracting its expected value and then dividing by its standard deviation. There are several reasons why you might want to standardize. Recall from Section 4.4 that the variance in the sum of two random variables that are not independent is the sum of their variances plus another term that measures the extent and direction of their dependency. The covariance of these two random variables is defined to be half the value of this term. When random variables are standardized, their covariance always falls between −1 and +1, which provides a uniform scale to indicate something about how dependent they are. Thus, we use the term, correlation, for the covariance of standardized random variables. Another reason why you may want to standardize random variables is to weight them more nearly equally, such as for combining different exam scores to determine class standing, or for combining different measurements into a single index.

Increase number of samples

To see another consequence of standardization, consider the values below:

STATEMENTS	$n = 16$		$n = 100$		$n = 1000$	
	$p = 1/4$	$p = 1/2$	$p = 1/4$	$p = 1/2$	$p = 1/4$	$p = 1/2$
sn# < −3	0.000	0.002	0.001	0.001	0.001	0.001
−3 ≤ sn# < −2	0.010	0.010	0.019	0.017	0.021	0.021
sn# = 0	0.225	0.196	0.084	0.078	0.000	0.000
0 <= sn# ≤ 1	0.180	0.297	0.280	0.325	0.341	0.341
3 < sn#	0.003	0.002	0.002	0.002	0.001	0.001

You can see what happens to different standardized binomial distributions as the number of samples, n, gets large. The values show the probability of some typical statements, using standardized binomial distributions for given values for n and p.

As n gets bigger, the distributions for different values for p get more similar to each other, and distributions for increasing values of n become more similar to each other. All distributions become close to one single distribution of a random variable often designated as z, whose probabilities can be calculated like this. First plot, over the horizontal t axis, the curve of

$$\text{Sqr}(2 \times \pi))^{-1} \times e^{-(t^2/2)}$$

in which $\pi = 3.14159$, as in the formula to calculate the area of a circle, "Sqr()" is a function that becomes the square root of its non-negative argument, and e = 2.71828, as in the Poisson formula. Now, $\Pr(x \leq z \leq y)$ is equal to the area under this curve between $t = x$ and $t = y$. Some of you may recognize this curve as the bell curve that represents the so-called "normal" distribution. It describes the normal distribution just as the horizontal line drawn over the unit interval at the height of 1 on the probability density axis describes the uniform distribution in Section 4.1.

Quick estimates

But what is so normal about it? Certainly its calculating rule is not normally convenient when it comes to actually trying to use it to calculate the probability of a statement. It has been made more convenient to use because its values have been pre-calculated and published in tables, which you can find in the backs of old statistics text books. There is also a rule of thumb that makes a normal distribution easy to use to approximate the 0.05 significance level of a test statistic if it is predicted to be normally distributed with known expected value and variance. Under these circumstances, the 0.05 significance is approximately two standard deviations away from the expected value.

Recall the observations of burrows on the north side of trees in Section 6.1; suppose you kept walking and observed seven more trees of which five had burrows on the north and two on the south. To use the binomial distribution you would have to calculate five terms and add them as before, but with 14 trees a normal distribution approximates the distribution predicted for the number with burrows on the north. Hypothesizing as before a probability of 1/2 that a burrow is on the north, the variance would be $14 \times 1/2 \times 1/2 = 7/2$, whose square root is about 15/8. Use this to estimate the 0.05 significance level to be the expected number (seven trees) plus twice the standard deviation, ($2 \times 15/8$ trees). If burrows were equally likely to be either side of a tree, you would observe 10 3/4 or more on the north of a tree with probability of about 0.05; 10 is not quite significant at 0.05.

What is so normal?

Note that the expression to calculate probabilities for the standard normal distribution does not contain p or n. At the limit, where n has become very large, the normal distribution does not depend on n or p. But the truly remarkable thing about the normal distribution is that it does not even depend on **b**, that binary random variable at the origin of all the randomness in the binomial distributions, **sn**. We could have started with any numerical valued random variable (except one so weird we can't even calculate its variance), call it **f**, and have used it in place of **b**. Add n independent samples of **f** and denote the sum with **fn**.

Standardize **fn#** = (**fn** − E(**fn**))/SQRT(V(**fn**)). The distribution of **fn#** also gets close to standard normal as n gets large. Thus, if a process can be construed as the sum of several nearly-the-same random processes happening independently, then the random variable it samples would be approximately normally distributed. For situations like this, e.g., wing size might be controlled additively by a large number of nearly independently recombining genes, a normal distribution really would be normal.

How to sample a normal distribution in a macro

Often classical statistics requires that you hypothesize normal distributions, but you might choose to when they seem appropriate. In such cases it will be useful for you to be able to sample a normal distribution in an EXCEL macro. After looking at the density distribution function above, it is not at all clear how to do this. Fortunately, a close approximation of the normal distribution can be sampled easily by arithmetically converting a sample of the uniformly distributed unit interval. I wrote this procedure to do it:

```
Sub NORMAL (X As Single)
    X = Rnd
    If (X >= 0.001) And (X <= 0.999) Then
        X = 0.603 * Log ( X / (1.0 - X) )
    Else
        If X > 0.999 Then
            X = 3.1
            End If
        If X < 0.001 Then
            X = -3.1
            End If
        End If ' (X >= ) And
    End Sub
```

These instructions illustrate the use of the function "Log()", which accepts a numerical argument and becomes its logarithm to the base e. The function "Log()" is not defined for 0; and when X contains 1 it generates a zero divide in the formula above. To avoid runtime errors, X is loaded directly with 3.1, the value a normal sample exceeds with probability 0.001. To convert the sample of a standardized normal distribution to one with mean u and variance v, multiply X by the square root of v and add u.

6.4   Negative binomial, Chi Square, and F distributions

Negative binomial

Binary, binomial, Poisson, normal, and uniform are names of parametric distributions, but there are many others. The negative binomial, like the binomial, is derived from a series of independent samples of a binary distribution and answers the question, What is the probability that I will have to observe exactly n samples of a binary random variable with $\Pr(\mathbf{b} = 1) = p$ to observe $\mathbf{b} = 1$ r times? The answer to this question is:

$$q^{((n-1)-(r-1))} \times p^{(r-1)} \times \frac{(n-1) \times (n-2) \times \ldots \times (n-r)}{(r-1) \times (r-2) \times \ldots \times 1} \times p$$

The first two factors are the probability of observing $r - 1$ times in some particular order during the first $n - 1$ samples $\mathbf{b} = 1$, and thus $\mathbf{b} = 0$ the remaining $n - (r - 1)$ times. The third factor is a quotient of products that calculates the number of such particular orders, and the last term is the probability of observing $\mathbf{b} = 1$ for sample n. Like the binomial, normal, and uniform distributions, this parametric distribution also has two parameters; they are p and r. The binary and Poisson have only one. A sample of the negative binomial distribution is a value for $\mathbf{n}$. To sample a negative binomial distribution computationally, it can be effective to pre-calculate, for the given values of the parameters p and r, the cumulative distribution $\Pr(\mathbf{n} = r)$, $\Pr(\mathbf{n} < r + 1)$, $\Pr(\mathbf{n} < r + 2)$, etc. for as many values as are relevant, and then use the statements shown earlier for sampling the Poisson distribution. To determine mathematically the expected value and variance of a negative binomial distribution requires taking infinite sums, which is beyond the scope of this text. It turns out that its expected value is $r \times p / (1 - p)$ and its variance is $r \times p / ((1 - p) \times (1 - p))$.

Chi Square and F

I mention here two other families of parametric distributions because they are common in classical statistics, and so you should be aware of them. However, they will probably not play a role in your hypotheses, if you take a computational approach to statistical argument. They are called Chi Square and F. You will have little use for them because they are not very plausible as hypothesized probability mechanisms for generating natural data; their role in classical statistics is to serve as the probability distributions predicted for test statistics arising from hypothesized probability mechanisms based on normal distributions. Because you calculate your own predicted probability distributions for your own test statistics, you probably will not need them in their classical role either. But it will be useful for you to understand them.

Chi Square is a random variable made by adding together a number of squared, standard, normally distributed random variables; the number added is called the degrees of freedom, which is the parameter for this one-parameter family of parametric distributions. Thus you could write a macro to estimate the distribution of Chi Square with one degree of freedom by sampling a standard normal distribution and squaring it, repeating this many times to make a bar graph. The amount by which a random sample of a normal distribution differs from its expected value is also normally distributed. Because it is mathematically convenient, squaring this difference is a common approach in classical statistics to measuring the extent to which a sample varies from its expected value. Thus the squared difference of a sample of a standard normal distribution from its mean is distributed as Chi Square with one degree of freedom. Chi Square distributions are often used to test how well quantities measured in the natural world (data) fit the distributions of random variables hypothesized to have generated them. We will examine this in more detail later, when we discuss estimation.

F is a two-parameter family of parametric distributions, derived from Chi Square; $F(m,n)$ is the ratio of a Chi Square with m degrees of freedom divided by a Chi Square with n degrees of freedom. The classical approach uses statistics derived from linear models, which we will discuss in the next chapter. These statistics are the ratios of two different ways to estimate variance from a small number of samples of a random variable. These estimates add the square of the deviation of samples of a random variable from its expected value. If the random variable has a normal distribution, then these sums will have Chi Square distributions, and their ratios F distributions.

There are many parametric distributions that will not concern us here. The classic text, Feller (1957), explains many of them. If you are interested, I suggest that you consult it.

6.5   Percentiles

In Chapter 4, I described the procedure SORT(L, TABLE()). It sorts from largest to smallest the array TABLE() of length L, often the L samples of a probability distribution that you have saved. I also described another procedure that calculated the heights of the bars in a bar graph showing the density of the distribution. It divided the theoretical range of the random variable being sampled, or if not known the observed range as evidenced by the first and last places in the now sorted TABLE(), into NSI equal-length intervals. Then it counted the number of samples in each interval. This approximates the density distribution with a bar graph, which shows the shape of a probability density distribution, especially its middle 90%. This is useful to train your intuition and to get familiar with probability distributions that you might want to use as data-generating mechanisms in your hypotheses. With your macros, you sample such distributions repeatedly as you compute a large number of simulated data sets. These samples result in simulated data sets from which you calculate simulated values of your test statistic. But 9 out of 10 of these values will fall in the middle 90% of the predicted probability distribution. For this reason, it is important to ensure that the basic shape of the middle of the distribution is appropriate to describe whatever variation you hypothesize as part of the causal mechanism. However, for rejecting a hypothesis, the tails of the distribution need to be estimated and reported very accurately.

Why percentiles?

A computational approach uses a hypothesized data-generating mechanism to predict a distribution for a test statistic. You have seen how a bar graph approximates the shape of a distribution. In the case of test statistics whose distributions are computationally predicted, it is not the middle, but the extremes of the predicted distribution that you want to estimate accurately and report in detail. It is the extreme 5% or so of the distribution that enables you to identify aspects of data that clearly contradict the hypothesis that predicted the distribution for the test statistic.

To identify the extreme thresholds of significance in a predicted distribution, you can describe the percentiles of a distribution. A percentile is a range of values that the test statistic will assume within a given percentage of the probability distribution density. For example, a test statistic might assume values between 2.375000 and 2.296296 with probabilities between the 4th and 5th percentile of the predicted distribution.

Interpreting percentiles

To make this more clear, I have written a macro to calculate the percentiles of any distribution. Below are the percentiles of a distribution simulated for MAD, the mean absolute deviation from the average inter-peak interval length, for the marine fossil data of Chapter 3. To demonstrate flexibility, MAD is slightly different from MSD, the test statistic we used there.

Maximum	Minimum	Sig. of minimum (%)	Maximum	Minimum	Sig. of minimum (%)
3.333333	2.897959	1	1.074380	1.020408	75
2.816327	2.666667	2	1.020000	0.962963	80
2.666667	2.500000	3	0.962963	0.911243	85*
2.500000	2.375000	4	0.906250	0.833333	90
2.375000	2.296296	5	0.833333	0.750000	95
2.296296	2.024691	10	0.750000	0.727273	96
2.000000	1.851852	15	0.727273	0.680000	97
1.840000	1.703704	20	0.677686	0.656250	98
1.702479	1.625000	25	0.650888	0.600000	99

The observed value for MAD is 0.9587. A small mean absolute deviation from average inter-peak interval length is evidence for a more regular cycling of ups and downs in the extinction rate of families of marine invertebrates over the past 500 million or so years. Because the data have provoked a controversy around this issue, it is not surprising that the observed value of MAD is somewhat low, but not too low. Its significance is about 0.18.

Look for its percentile, marked with *, near the bottom of the table of percentiles, and find it in the interval representing the percentiles between 80% and 85% rather closer to the 80% threshold. Because the small values hold the significance for this particular argument, we subtract these percentages from 100% to get a significance in the 15% to 20% range. One simulated estimate of realized significance for the observed value of MAD was about 0.187, which is consistent with the percentiles reported here.

Such a table of percentiles is similar to the tables of the percentiles of the pre-calculated distributions you can find in the backs of old statistics books. For distributions of continuing interest, I write percentiles to a worksheet so that I can consult them again at a later time. You can compute tailor-made realized significances of simple and specifically focused test statistics whenever you need them, so why ever consult tables of percentiles, the old fashioned way? Sometimes you may want to simulate a predicted probability distribution before any data have been observed. Also, if you do not have an observed value of your test statistic to compare then you cannot increment counters, like SIGHI and SIGLO, to estimate realized significance directly.

A macro to calculate percentiles

I wrote the macro PERCENTILES(L, TABLE()) to discover and write the percentiles for MAD shown above. First I called SORT(NOS, DISTR()) to arrange in order the NOS simulated values of the test statistic saved in the array DISTR(). The procedure PERCENTILES(L, TABLE()) loads in place K the number of samples in a single percentile range. The first K places in DIST() represent the 1% percentile. DISTR(1) and DISTR(K) hold the maximum and minimum values of MAD for the 1% percentile. The minimum value is the 1% significance threshold. The next K places, DISTR(K+1) to DISTR(2×K) represent the 2% percentile, as do successive blocks of K places for successive percentiles. The max and min values for MAD, and their percentile, are reported for the five single percentiles on the tails of the distribution. From 5% to 25% these are reported in 5% intervals, and the middle half of the distribution is not even reported.

This is my procedure PERCENTILES; DISTR must be already sorted:

```
Sub PERCENTILES(NOS As Integer, DISTR() As Single)
Dim NR,K,T,I,R,J As Integer
Worksheets("Sheet1").Cells(1,1) = "Max"
Worksheets("Sheet1").Cells(1,2) = "Min"
Worksheets("Sheet1").Cells(1,3) = "Sig"
NR = NOS
K = 0
Do Until NR <= 0 'Discover # samples in 1%
   K = K + 1
   NR = NR - 100
   Loop 'Until NR <= 0
```

```
T = 0
For I = 1 To 5 'write high tail 5 x 1% intervals
    Worksheets("Sheet1").Cells(I+1,1) = DISTR(T+1)
    Worksheets("Sheet1").Cells(I+1,2) = DISTR(T+K)
    Worksheets("Sheet1").Cells(I+1,3) = DISTR(I)
    T = T + K
    Next I
R = K * 5 '5% intervals
J = 5
For I = 1 To 18 'write middle 0.90
    J = J + 5
    Worksheets("Sheet1").Cells(I+7,1) = DISTR(T+1)
    Worksheets("Sheet1").Cells(I+7,2) = DISTR(T+R)
    Worksheets("Sheet1").Cells(I+7,3) = DISTR(J)
    T = T + R
    Next I
For I = 1 To 5 'write low tail 5 x 1% intervals
    J = J + 1
    Worksheets("Sheet1").Cells(I+26,1) = DISTR(T+1)
    Worksheets("Sheet1").Cells(I+26,2) = DISTR(T+K)
    Worksheets("Sheet1").Cells(I+26,3) = DISTR(J)
    T = T + k
    Next I
End Sub 'PERCENTILES
```

Quit while you are ahead

Sometimes it is expensive to collect data. A very old statistical error is quit while you are ahead. Mendel, counting his famous peas, made this error. He kept making observations until his results looked convincing; he needed convincing-looking results because he did not have the help of modern classical statistics. By modern standards, his results are too good to be statistically plausible. If you do not use your data to calculate the distribution predicted for your test statistic, percentiles reporting the tails of the distribution predicted for your test statistic will be independent of the data you later gather.

7 | Linear model

7.1 Linear model

Fundamental to observing phenomena, hypothesizing explanations, and arguing their differential credibility is the recognition and quantification of distinctions. Are things different? If so, how different are they? The question, Can we distinguish by their weight the two groups of fish caught on different dry flies?, is an example. We have discussed several test statistics relevant to this question. Now we will examine an approach used by classical statistics to address the same basic question. This approach to hypothesis formation is widely used in the published literature of every natural science, and is not uncommon in the more quantitative publications of social science as well. It will be important for you to understand it, and possibly even use it, in your own work.

This approach is to hypothesize a non-probabilistic causal mechanism; any variation in the observed data that is not accounted for by this mechanism is attributed to error. This error is construed as random, quantified in a particular way that was convenient when people had to compute without computers. These non-probabilistic hypotheses are actually a whole family of such hypotheses, called the linear model. From this family, the particular member that minimizes the random (unexplained) variability in the data attributed to error is chosen. The result is a description of the variability in your data, and several candidates for test statistics.

The classical approach

Classical statistics goes on to hypothesize a particular mechanism that samples a normally distributed random variable to generate error, and defines some more complicated test statistics whose predicted probability distributions have been pre-calculated. As discussed earlier, the probability distributions predicted for some of these test statistics are the ratio of two

Chi Square distributions, which is called the F distribution. At this point, however, these constraints cease to be useful. Once you understand how the linear model structures data and suggests a few test statistics, you can use a computational approach to hypothesize probability mechanisms and discover distributions for test statistics predicted by them.

To follow, I first discuss concepts of quantifying error, then I describe the non-probabilistic hypotheses, and explain the techniques for minimizing error to choose a particular member of the linear model family. Because error-minimizing techniques use linear algebra, the whole approach was named linear model, but this is a misnomer, because the function relating the causes to the effects is not linear, in the mathematical sense in which, for example, expected value is linear. Finally I discuss a generalization of the approach to a wider class of scientific questions, which is called linear regression.

7.2   Quantifying error

Ways to quantify error

Fundamental to quantifying error is the notion that a single number represents several numbers. For example, suppose you counted the number of seeds in each of six Varyberry fruits. You got these counts: 0 1 2 4 4 7.

You chose 4 as a single number to represent all six numbers. One way to evaluate how good a job 4 does as a representative of all six numbers is to measure how much error results when you use 4 instead of the real measurements.

One possible measure is the number of times 4 is wrong. In this case, 4 is wrong for four fruits and right for two fruits. By this measure, any other number would be wrong for more fruits, so 4 is the best. But some of the errors that 4 makes are bigger than others.

These are the errors: 4 3 2 0 0 3. They are the absolute (ignoring the sign) deviations from 4. So another possible way to measure how much error results when you use 4 instead of the real measurements is to Sum the Absolute Deviations, called SAD. By this criterion, the error made by 4 is 12. According to SAD, is 4 the best representative? According to SAD, how much error results when you use 2 instead of 4? What representative number(s) makes the minimum error, i.e., minimizes SAD? Maybe the best representative (by this criterion) is not even one of the observed seed numbers. How much error results when you use 3 as the representative? Is it really a tie, or do you think that 3 is better than 4?

Perhaps you think big errors are worse than little errors. You could square all the errors before adding them up. This sum of squared errors, SSE, would make big errors contribute proportionally more to the total error than little errors. By this criterion you would choose a representative number that made bigger little errors in order to make littler big errors. By this criterion 4 results in an SSE of 38. What SSE results when you use 3?

Suppose you quantified error using the sum of the square roots of the errors, instead of the squares. The bigger the error, the less important the next increment of error becomes. You might have a situation in which you recognize that there might be a few atypical observations, but you would like the representative to be close to most of them. This criterion would pick out a representative nearer 2, recognizing the fruit with seven seeds as atypical.

Suppose instead of square roots, you took 100th roots. What does this mean? Any errors that were not 0 would become close to 1, so this criterion would count the number of times the representative is wrong. I started this discussion of quantifying error with this "a miss is as good as a mile!" criterion, which selected 4 as the representative.

What about the sum of the errors each raised to the 100th power? The biggest error makes up most of that sum. So this criterion, a miss is as good as a mile, chooses the representative that minimizes the biggest error, which would be 3 1/2 in the Varyberry example above.

Sum of squared error

From among all these choices, and others not mentioned, classical statistics uses SSE as a way to measure error, in part because it makes it easier to manipulate the complicated math. To illustrate this I will show you how to find a/the representative that minimizes the sum of squared error. I could write a macro that incremented through the range of possibilities computing SSE for each, but that would be too computational for the classical tradition. Instead, use abstract reasoning, like this. Denote with r a candidate representative, with $SSE(r)$ the sum of squared error that would be made if r were the representative, and denote with $o[i]$ the ith of n observations.

Now write:

$$SSE(r) = (r - o[1])^2 + (r - o[2])^2 + \ldots + (r - o[n])^2$$

and use calculus to find the r that makes $SSE(r)$ smallest. The derivative with respect to r is:

$$d(SSE(r))/dr = 2 \times r - 2 \times o[1] + 2 \times r - 2 \times o[2] + \ldots + 2 \times r - 2 \times o[n]$$

which we set equal to 0:

$$0 = 2 \times n * r - 2(o[1] + o[2] + \ldots + o[n])$$

Now solve for r to get:

$$r = (o[1] + o[2] + \ldots + o[n])/n$$

which we call the average of the observed counts.

So, it turns out that the average minimized SSE. Thus, another way to define the average is as the representative number that minimizes the sum of squared error. To many of us it seems natural to choose the average to represent the whole group, which is another reason why SSE is appealing as an error criterion. Besides, as we saw above, SAD can't always make up its mind.

Choose a linear model with SSE

We can use SSE as a minimizing criterion to choose a member of the linear model family of hypotheses whenever we have a distinction (the cause) and we have measured several of the things distinguished (the effect). To illustrate this in concrete terms, suppose you have counted the number of seeds (effects) in each of several fruits from two different Varyberry bushes, call them bush 0 and bush 1 (which bush is the cause). For each fruit you have two numbers: the number of the bush where you collected the fruit and the number of seeds in that fruit. Do the two different bushes produce fruits with (i.e., cause) different numbers of seeds? Could we distinguish the bushes based on the numbers of seeds in their fruits? The linear model hypothesis suggests that we could at least partially distinguish the bushes if they produced fruits with different average numbers of seeds.

To express the linear model hypothesis, denote with Y(*i*) the number of seeds in the *i*th fruit of the *n* fruits whose seeds were counted, and with X(*i*) the number of the bush from which it came.

The family of linear-model hypotheses states that the number of seeds Y(*i*) in fruit *i*, caused by the bush X(*i*) that grew it, is some number of seeds, denoted B0, plus some additional number of seeds determined by the product of X(*i*) times some other number denoted B1. The number of seeds observed might differ from the number of seeds theoretically caused by the linear model. This difference is called error. The amount of error associated with fruit *i* is denoted E(*i*). Using this notation, we can write:

$$Y(i) = B0 + B1 \times X(i) + E(i)$$

If we subtract the number caused from the number we observed then we get the signed error, E(*i*) = Y(*i*) – (B0 + B1 × X(*i*)), which is positive if this guess were too small and negative if this guess were too big.

This linear model is a family of hypotheses that describe a relationship between the cause (which bush) and the effects (number of seeds in a fruit). This family has two parameters, B0 and B1. According to the linear model idea, the best description of this relationship is made by the member of the family that minimizes the sum of squared errors. This member is found by finding values for B0 and B1 that minimize the sum over all fruits of E(*i*) × E(*i*). I will show you how to do this in the next section.

7.3   Linear model in matrix form

SSE(B0,B1)

The task at this point is to choose numerical values for B0 and B1 so that Y(*i*) = B0 + B1 × X() + E(*i*) becomes the deterministic hypothesis that X(*i*) causes Y(*i*) and that makes the sum of the squared errors minimum. It is helpful to remember in the manipulations to follow that the distinction represented by the X(*i*)s and the measurements represented by the Y(*i*)s have all been made, and now are fixed, known facts. What can vary are the numbers B0 and B1. Some choices of B0 and B1 will be better than others, i.e., make smaller errors. We use the sum of squared errors to make precise this concept of better and worse values of B0 and B1. Thus, we want to choose values for B0 and B1 that result in a sum of squared errors that is smaller than for any other choice. First, we denote SSE(B0,B1) to indicate that its value depends on the variable numerical values for B0 and B1. Then we write an expression for SSE(B0,B1) that indicates how we would calculate it. Next we take its derivatives with respect to B0 and B1 and set each of these equal to zero to get two simultaneous equations; and finally solve these equations to get calculating formulas for B0 and B1. This is the expression for SSE(B0,B1), in which ! = means equal by definition:

$$(Y[1] - (B0 + B1 \times X(1)))^2 + \ldots + (Y[n] - (B0 + B1 \times X(n)))^2$$
$$! = \sum_i^n (Y(i) - (B0 + B1 \times X(i)))^2$$

Multiply out the squares:

$$= \sum_i^n (Y(i)^2 - 2 \times Y(i) \times (B0 + B1 \times X(i)) + (B0 + B1 \times X(i))^2)$$
$$= \sum_i^n (Y(i)^2 - 2 \times Y(i) + B0^2 + 2 \times B0 \times B1 \times X(i) + B1^2 \times X(i)^2)$$

Now take the derivatives with respect to B0 and B1:

$$dSSE(B0, B1)/dB0 = \sum_i^n (-2 \times Y(i) + 2 \times B0 \times 2 \times B1 \times X(i))$$

$$dSSE(B0, B1)/dB1 = \sum_i^n (-2 \times Y(i) \times X(i) + 2 \times B0 \times X(i) + 2 \times B1 \times X(i)^2)$$

Set these two derivatives each equal to zero and rearrange to get:

$$\sum_i^n (Y(i) - (B0 + B1 \times X(i))) \times 1 = 0 \tag{7.1}$$

$$\sum_i^n (Y(i) - (B0 + B1 \times X(i))) \times X(i) = 0$$

A look at some matrices

For now we will leave Equations 7.1, and consider them again after we have looked at some matrices.

Denote with B the column vector of the two numbers B0 and B1

$$B = \begin{pmatrix} B0 \\ B1 \end{pmatrix}$$

The X matrix shown below has a column of 1s and a column to indicate the context of each observation. It is called the design matrix. In the equation below, it is preceded by its transpose:

$$\begin{pmatrix} 1 & 1 & \cdots 1 \\ X(1) & X(2) \cdots X(n) \end{pmatrix} \begin{pmatrix} 1 & X(1) \\ 1 & X(2) \\ \cdot & \cdot \\ \cdot & \cdot \\ 1 & X(n) \end{pmatrix} = \begin{pmatrix} \sum_i^n 1 & \sum_i^n X(i) \\ \sum_i^n X(i) & \sum_i^n X(i)^2 \end{pmatrix}$$

$$X^T \qquad \times \qquad X \qquad = \qquad \text{Matrix} \qquad (7.2)$$

Denote with Y the column vector of observed seed counts:

$$\begin{pmatrix} 1 & 1 & \cdots 1 \\ X(1) & X(2) \cdots X(n) \end{pmatrix} \begin{pmatrix} Y(1) \\ Y(2) \\ \cdot \\ \cdot \\ Y(n) \end{pmatrix} = \begin{pmatrix} \sum_i^n Y(i) \\ \sum_i^n X(i) \times Y(i) \end{pmatrix}$$

$$X^T \qquad \times \quad Y$$

This enables you to write the following matrix expression:

$$\begin{pmatrix} \sum_i^n B0 & + \sum_i^n X(i) \times B1 \\ \sum_i^n X(i) \times B0 & + \sum_i^n X(i)^2 \times B1 \end{pmatrix} - \begin{pmatrix} \sum_i^n Y(i) \\ \sum_i^n X(i) \times Y(i) \end{pmatrix}$$

$$X^T \times X \times B \qquad - \qquad X^T \times Y$$

Doing the subtraction and combining the sums gives:

$$\begin{pmatrix} \sum_i^n (Y(i) - (B0 + B1 \times X(i))) \times 1 \\ \sum_i^n (Y(i) - (B0 + B1 \times X(i))) \times X(i) \end{pmatrix}$$

Solve the matrix equation

Compare this with the Equations 7.1 to see that the values for B0 and B1 that minimize the sum of squared error are the solution for the vector B in the matrix equation:

$$X^T \times X \times B - X^T \times Y = 0.$$

Solving gives an important formula

$$B = (X^T \times X)^{-1} \times (X^T \times Y) \tag{7.3}$$

The inverse of the product of the transpose of the design matrix times the design matrix itself is denoted C and called the variance-covariance matrix. When there is one design variable, C is a 2×2 matrix. You may remember from high school:

$$\begin{pmatrix} a & b \\ c & d \end{pmatrix}^{-1} = \frac{1}{ad - bc} \begin{pmatrix} d & -b \\ -c & a \end{pmatrix} \tag{7.4}$$

You can use Equation 7.4 to invert Matrix 7.2 to calculate C.

Use the solution

To use Equation 7.3 to calculate B0 and B1 in our Varyberry example, denote with $n0$ and $n1$ the number of fruits collected from bush 0 and bush 1 respectively. Now $n = n0 + n1$.

$$\sum_i^n X(i) = n1$$

Remember that $X(i)$ is the bush number of fruit i.

Use Equation 7.1 and Matrix 7.2 to calculate C, and then Equation 7.3 to calculate values of B0 and B1 in our example:

$$
\begin{bmatrix} B0 \\ B1 \end{bmatrix} = \begin{bmatrix} 1/n0 & -1/n0 \\ -1/n0 & (n0 + n1)/(n0 \times n1) \end{bmatrix} \begin{bmatrix} \sum_i^n Y(i) \\ \sum_i^n X(i) \times Y(i) \end{bmatrix}
$$

$$
B \quad = \qquad\qquad C \qquad\qquad \times \qquad X^T \times Y
$$

The indicated algebraic manipulations show that B0 is the average seeds/fruit in bush 0 (call it A0) and that B1 is A1 (the average seeds/fruit in bush 1) minus A0.

$$
\text{Thus,} \quad \begin{pmatrix} B0 \\ B1 \end{pmatrix} = \begin{pmatrix} A0 \\ A1 - A0 \end{pmatrix}
$$

For the Varyberry example, the specific linear model hypothesis is: $Y(i) = A0 + (A1 - A0) \times X(i)$, which states that the bush on which the fruit grew caused the average number of seeds among fruits on that bush, and we call error any deviations from this caused amount. All this manipulation and reasoning came up with an intuitively reasonable result, which is reassuring. However, I could have made a simpler case for choosing the within-bush average to represent that part of the seed number caused by the bush; within-bush average minimizes squared error. Why bother with all of this?

Why bother with matrices?

In this example, the $X(i)$ values represent only two different bushes. This was done to keep the algebraic manipulations more accessible, so it would be easier to follow the reasoning. However, the results of these manipulations are equally valid for $X(i)$s that assume many different numerical values. For example, $X(i)$ could be a measurement, such as the length of fruit i. We still think of such measurements $X(i)$ as representing a cause or a basis to explain the variability in the measurements $Y(i)$, but unlike within-bush average, in cases like these Equation 7.3 comes up with values for B0 and B1 that are not at all so easy to compute in other ways.

To be mathematically more correct, Equation 7.3 works only for a design matrix, X, for which the inverse matrix:

$$
(X^T \times X)^{-1} = C
$$

exists. When it makes sense to put the $X(i)$s on an axis of real numbers, the numbers $Y(i)$ can be placed on a perpendicular axis, and the things that were measured can be plotted on two axes at co-ordinates $(X(i), Y(i))$. In this case, B0 is the intercept and B1 the slope of the straight line with least squared error, where for each observation i, error, $E(i)$, is the distance from $Y(i)$ to that line, measured parallel to the Y axis.

Thus, a linear model gives us a description of one way a straight line can attribute deterministic cause, characterized by three numbers, B0 the intercept, B1 the slope, and SSE the sum of squared errors. When we include a random process with this deterministic hypothesis, B0, B1, and SSE can all become potentially interesting test statistics.

7.4   Using a linear model

Use Equation 7.3

You collected five Varyberry fruits at different heights above or below the middle of the bush, and counted the number of seeds in each fruit. These are your data.

Fruit index	1	2	3	4	5
Height	-2	-1	0	1	2
Number of seeds	0	0	1	1	3

You hypothesize that height determines seed number except for some error, according to a linear model. To write this, fruit index is represented by i, height of fruit i by $X(i)$, and number of seeds in fruit i by $Y(i)$. The column of all five height values is represented by X and the column of all five seed counts by Y. Now you can write:

$$Y(i) = B0 + B1 \times X(i) + E(i) \tag{7.5}$$

This equation hypothesizes that X (height) is the cause, and Y (number of seeds) is what it causes. Y is sometimes called the response. E the error has a value that depends on which fruit, so it too is a column of numbers, of which the ith is $E(i)$. We can calculate B0 and B1 using important formula Equation 7.3 like this:

$$Y^T = (0, \ 0, \ 1, 1, 3) \qquad \text{and}$$

$$X^T = \begin{pmatrix} 1, & 1, & 1, & 1, & 1 \\ -2, & -1, & 0, & 1, & 2 \end{pmatrix}. \qquad \text{Thus, } C = \begin{pmatrix} 1/5 & 0 \\ 0 & 1/10 \end{pmatrix}$$

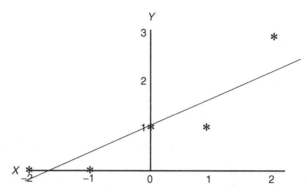

Figure 7.1 Graph of the linear model, $Y = 0.7 * X + 1.0 + E$. The plot of height, X, and the number of seeds, Y, is shown with * for each of the five fruits

$$X^T \times Y = \begin{pmatrix} 5 \\ 7 \end{pmatrix} \qquad B = C \times X^T \times Y = \begin{pmatrix} 1 \\ 7/10 \end{pmatrix}$$

Substitute these values for B0 and B1 into the general hypothesis, Equation 7.5 above, to get the specific hypothesis $Y(i) = 1 + 7/10 \times X(i) + E(i)$. This says that the number of seeds in a fruit is determined by 7/10 times the height of the fruit plus one seed, plus some error.

Plot the linear model

If we ignore the error for the time being, then the values for X and Y that would make the hypothesis exactly true plot as a straight line on a two-dimensional graph with an X axis and a Y axis, as shown in Figure 7.1. In Figure 7.1, the data points are shown with *. The vertical distance up or down from any * to this line indicates the error for that data point. Among all possible straight lines that could have been drawn with these axes, the sum of the squares of the distances parallel to the Y axis from the data points to the line is least for this line. For this reason, this line is sometimes called the least squares regression of seed number on height. The term, regression, comes from an old-fashioned calculating algorithm, and not from what the line is conceptually.

Calculate SSE – In this example the errors (sometimes called residuals) are: 0.4, –0.3, 0.0, –0.7, 0.6 . The sum of their squares is:

$$\sum_{i}^{5} (E(i) \times E(i)) = 0.16 + 0.09 + 0.0 + 0.49 + 0.36 = 1.10 = SSE$$

More matrix algebra, which I will not belabor, demonstrates that:

$$SSE = Y^T \times Y - B \times X^T \times Y$$

With this formula you can calculate the sum of squared error for the hypothesis that minimizes it, once B has been calculated using important formula Equation 7.3. SSE tells you how bad the "best" hypothesis is. Use this formula to calculate from the data the sum of squared error in the least squares linear regression. This line hypothesizes how the height above the ground determines the number of seeds in a fruit. The calculations look like this:

$$SSE = Y^T \times Y - B \times X^T \times Y = 11.0 - 9.9 = 1.1$$

If you ignore fruit height then you can summarize seeds per fruit with the average number of seeds in a fruit, which is 1. In this case the sum of squared error is 6, which is denoted SSE0. So observing the fruit height and using it in a linear model to predict the seed number with a least squared straight line reduces the sum of squared error by 6.0 − 1.1 = 4.9, which is 81.7% of 6.0. We say that the linear model (or the line) explains 81.7% of the squared error.

Sub LINMO

To calculate the least squares hypothesis in the family $Y(i) = b0 + b1 \times X(i) + error(i)$ of linear models that minimizes squared error, I wrote this macro procedure, called LINMO.

```
Sub LINMO (L As Integer, X() As Single, Y() As Single, B0 As
    Single, B1 As Single, SSE As Single, SSE0 As Single)
    'The 2 lines above should be on 1 line in your macro editor
    'Y(I) = B0 + B1 * X(I) + error(I)
    'LINMO finds B0 and B1 that minimize sum squared errors, SSE
Dim D, SY, SXTY, XBAR, YBAR As Single
Dim C(4) As Single
Dim I, K As Integer
    'calculate C, the varcovar matrix of B0 and B1 for design, X
    'C(1) = C(1,1) C(2) =C(1,2) C(3) =C(2,1) C(4) =C(2,2)
C(1) = 0
```

```
C(2) = 0
For I = 1 To L
   C(1) = C(1) + X(I) * X(I)
   C(2) = C(2) + X(I)
   Next I
C(3) = C(2)
C(4) = L
D = 1 / (C(4) * C(1) - C(2) * C(3)) 'determinant
C(1) = C(1) * D
C(2) = -C(2) * D
C(3) = -C(3) * D
                                      T
C(4) = C(4) * D          'C now contains (X * X) inverse}

XBAR = 0
YBAR = 0

SY = 0
SXTY = 0      'Initialize sum of x times y

For I = 1 To L
   XBAR = XBAR + X(I)
   SY = SY + Y(I)
   SXTY = SXTY + X(I) * Y(I)
   Next I
XBAR = XBAR / L
YBAR = SY / L
B0 = C(1) * SY + C(2) * SXTY                    'intercept
B1 = C(3) * SY + C(4) * SXTY                       'slope
SSE = 0                    'calculate sum squared errors
SSE0 = 0

For I = 1 To L
   SSE = SSE + Y(I) * Y(I)
   SSE0 = SSE0 + (YBAR - Y(I)) * (YBAR - Y(I))
   Next I
SSE = SSE - (B0 * SY + B1 * SXTY)
End Sub
```

Test Sub LINMO

To test and later use this procedure I wrote a macro that reads from a worksheet the number of observed cases and the value of X and Y for each one, calls LINMO, and writes results back to the worksheet. I designed the worksheet to have the number of cases in cell (1,1), a column of Xs starting in row 3 of column 1, and a column of corresponding Ys starting in row 3 of column 2. The resulting B0, B1, SSE0, and SSE were written in columns 2 through 5 of row 1, and the caused values of Y (YHAT) and their errors in columns 3 and 4 starting in row 3. My macro looks like this:

```
Sub CALLINMO()
Dim X(10) As Single
Dim Y(10) As Single
Dim YHAT(10) As Single
Dim R, N As Integer
Dim SSE0 As Single      'Places in the computer's memory that
Dim SSE As Single       'you pass in the calling sequence
Dim B0 As Single        'of a procedure need to be "Dim-ed"
Dim B1 As Single        'each on their own line in some versions
MsgBox ("Run CALLIMNO")
N = Worksheets("Sheet1").Cells(1, 1) 'Number of cases
For R = 1 To N
  X(R) = Worksheets("Sheet1").Cells(R + 2, 1)
  Y(R) = Worksheets("Sheet1").Cells(R + 2, 2)
  Next R
Call LINMO(N, X(), Y(), B0, B1, SSE, SSE0)
     'Calling sequence must be in the same order as defined above
Worksheets("Sheet1").Cells(1, 2) = B0      'Write results
Worksheets("Sheet1").Cells(1, 3) = B1
Worksheets("Sheet1").Cells(1, 4) = SSE0
Worksheets("Sheet1").Cells(1, 5) = SSE
For R = 1 To N
  YHAT(R) = B0 + X(R) * B1
  Worksheets("Sheet1").Cells(R + 2, 3) = YHAT(R)
  Worksheets("Sheet1").Cells(R + 2, 4) = Y(R) - YHAT(R)
  Next R
MsgBox ("End LINMO")
End Sub
```

When run with the Varyberry data, my worksheet looks like this:

5	1	0.7	6	1.1
−2	0	−0.4	0.4	
−1	0	0.3	−0.3	
0	1	1.0	0.0	
1	1	1.7	−0.7	
2	3	2.4	0.6	

If EXCEL does not format the number of decimal places you want, highlight the cells, bring down the format menu, select format cells, select "Number" and then choose the number of decimal places you want.

7.5   Hypotheses of random for a linear model

Statistical hypotheses include a concept of random

So far in this discussion of linear models, I have not yet considered any random mechanisms to include in a linear-model hypothesis. To test a hypothesis statistically it must be able to predict a probability distribution for a test statistic. Thus, a statistical hypothesis must also specify a concept of random. To take a computational approach, that concept of random is used to generate data sets with the same structure as those observed; the value of a test statistic is calculated from 1000 or more such simulated data sets to estimate the probability distribution predicted for the test statistic. All that mathematical notation, manipulation, and argument in the previous section made a linear model that just structures and describes data in terms of a deterministic cause and its error. If the experimental design, X, includes more than one context, then least squared error always specifies a particular member of the linear model family of deterministic hypotheses; there are always a B0 and a B1 so that $Y = B0 + B1 \times X + E$ results in minimum squared error. A linear model would produce a deterministic hypothesis even in cases when X did not cause Y. To test whether the variability in X determines more of the variability in Y than it would at random, a concept of random must be included in the hypothesis.

Null hypothesis

One way I can test a linear model is to hypothesize that X does not cause Y. I would state such a hypothesis in terms of a random variable to generate data, and choose a test statistic to quantify something relevant. I would state my hypothesis explicitly enough to use it to write a macro to simulate a data set. That data set would be an example of what might have been observed in the context of the random variation hypothesized under the so-called null hypothesis that X did not cause Y. When I use that simulated data set to calculate a value for my test statistic, it samples the probability distribution of that test statistic predicted by the hypothesis that simulated the data set.

Perhaps you have already recognized that the question of two Varyberry bushes, each bearing several fruits with observed varying numbers of seeds, and the question of two dry flies each catching several fish of varying weights, are structurally the same. In the specific linear-model hypothesis for two Varyberry bushes, B0 is the average number of seeds in fruits from bush 0 and B1 is (the average number of seeds in fruits from bush 1) minus (the average number of seeds in fruits from bush 0). In the case that $X(i)$ is 0, fruit i is from bush 0, so $Y(i) = B0 + B1 \times 0 + E(i) = B0 + E(i)$. This confirms that $Y(i)$ = bush 0 average + fruit i error. If $X(i)$ is 1 then fruit i is from bush 1. Evaluate the same formula for $X(i) = 1$ to confirm that $Y(i)$ = bush 1 average + fruit i error. In this way, each bush determines its own average number of seeds. The B1 parameter is the difference of these averages. Even though we did not use the difference of the averages when comparing weights of fish caught on different flies, it was one of the test statistics discussed.

Test statistics for a linear model

Now I will use B1 as a test statistic and borrow from Chapter 5 the idea for a hypothesis that the number of seeds in a fruit is determined by sampling the SAME random variable no matter on which bush the fruit grows. If the B1 calculated from the observed data is improbably large according to the probability distribution predicted for B1 by this hypothesis, then that will argue that different random variables determine seed number for each of the two bushes.

The hypothesis that the number of seeds in a fruit from bush 0 samples the same random variable as does the number of seeds in a fruit from bush 1 predicts that the expected value of B1 is 0. The expected values of the number of seeds in a fruit are the same for both bushes because the same random variable (with the same distribution) is determining seed number in each bush. The linear-model deterministic hypothesis states that if B1 is not calculated to be 0 then bush identity participates to determine seed number. The statistical hypothesis above states that B1 is really zero, but may end up with a non-zero value from the least-squares calculating process as a consequence of sampling the variation in the single random variable that determines seed number in the same way for each bush. The probability distribution predicted for B1 describes the variation B1 would have if its observed value was just a consequence of this random process.

This statistical hypothesis states that B1 is actually 0, so in linear model notation: $Y(i) = B0 + E(i)$. Recall that the average is the representative that minimizes squared error. Thus the value for this B0 that minimizes squared error is the average seed number among the fruits pooled from both bushes; this sum of the squared errors is the SSE0 earlier discussed. Because the sum of squared error is usually reduced and never increased by any distinction, even a bogus one, SSE ≤ SSE0. Basically, this statistical hypothesis states that the distinction into two bushes IS bogus as far as number of seeds in a fruit is concerned. The difference SSE0 − SSE is an artifact of sampling the variation in the single random variable that determines seed number in the same way for each bush. Thus it becomes apparent that SSE0 − SSE is also a relevant test statistic. The probability distribution predicted for SSE0 − SSE describes the variation it would have if it were just the result of such random sampling.

Concepts of random for linear models

There are many reasonable ways to define a probability distribution for the random variable that describes the variation in seed number, hypothesized to be the same for each bush. One way is to re-sample the numbers of seeds observed in the fruits pooled from both bushes, as in Chapter 5. Once you have defined that random variable, you can write a macro to sample it as many times as you have observed real fruits to create a simulated data set, which provides a simulated column vector Y. Use Y in important formula Equation 7.3 to calculate a sample of the distribution predicted for B1, or any other relevant test statistic. Your macro does this a thousand times or more, each time comparing the observed value of the test statistic with a simulated value and incrementing the significance counters, SIGHI and SIGLO. If you want, save the simulated values in a table and then sort and plot the distribution as a bar graph, or in percentiles, to report the predicted probability distribution.

With the exception of important formula Equation 7.3, you could do all of this already by the end of Chapter 5. In the case of two Varyberry bushes, and more generally any two or more groups, you do not even need Equation 7.3 because you know that within-group averages minimize squared error, so you can calculate the sum of squared errors directly. In any case, looking at these examples of two groups as linear models is instructive for several reasons.

Examples are instructive

In the two-groups examples, you know what the answers are already, so when you use important formula Equation 7.3 and get the same answers, it inspires your confidence and trains your intuition. The two-groups example simplifies somewhat the notation used in the arguments that manipulate that notation so that it is easier for you to follow those arguments. However, important formula Equation 7.3 still holds when the design matrix does not have just group labels, but instead values of experimentally controlled, or observed, variables in the role of possible causes. In such cases important formula Equation 7.3 really is important to calculate B0, B1, and SSE. The hypothesis that B1 is zero, and consequently the Xs do not really participate in determining the Ys, can still apply with the same logic. In this case, B0 is not trivial and can also be used as a test statistic along with B1 and sums or ratios of various squared errors.

ANOVA

Even when the Xs are just group codes and we know that the Bs will turn out to be within-group averages, calculating sums of squared errors around within-group averages, and around pooled-group averages, and then doing more arithmetic with them to calculate a statistic with a pre-calculated distribution, is all part of an important technique of classical statistics called Analysis of Variance, or ANOVA for short. As is often the case, it is named not for what it tests, but for how you calculate the test statistic, which is a ratio of two estimates of variance. If other conditions are met and there are enough data, this ratio approximates a distribution family called F. We will not use the restrictive hypothesis and complicated test statistics cleverly conceived by classical statistics for ANOVA data structures. However, those data structures and the scientific questions that go with them are interesting and relevant.

Consider again the Varyberry data of Section 7.3. To test the linear- model hypothesis that fruit height explains some of the variation in the number of seeds in a fruit, you need to choose a test statistic and to hypothesize a random variable to describe the variation, if fruit height did not contribute to determining number of seeds. You could choose the slope of the regression line, B1, as your test statistic, and re-sample the number of seeds to make the single random variable that all fruit heights sample.

A macro to calculate the predicted distribution of B1

To write a macro to do this you could enlarge the CALLINMO() macro of the previous section. You need to name places to pool seed numbers, to randomly sample this pool, to put the value of simulated B1, and to count high and low realized significances. Below is my design sketch of a macro to do this:

```
Sub FRUITHEIGHT()
    'Looks like CALLINMO but includes the following place name
    Dim POOL(5), X As Single
    Dim J, NS, SIGHI As Integer
    Dim SB1 As Single
    *** all the rest of CALLINMO down to last MsgBox ***
    MsgBox("Begin Simulations")

    For R = 1 To N
        POOL(R) = Y(R)
    Next R
    SIGHI = 0
    'SIGLO is not really relevant to this question
    Randomize
```

```
For NS = 1 To 1000
  For R = 1 To N
    X = Rnd * N
    J = 1
    Do Until J > X
      J = J + 1
    Loop
    Y(R) = POOL(J)
    Next R
    Call LINMO(N,X(),Y(),B0,SB1,SSE,SSE0)
    If SB1 >= B1 Then
      SIGHI = SIGHI + 1
    End If
  Next NS
  Worksheets("Sheet1").Cells(1,6) = SIGHI
  MsgBox("End FRUITHEIGHT")
End Sub 'FRUITHEIGHT
```

7.6   Two-way analysis of variance

Example data

Big fry are 5 cm long and small fry are 1 cm long. They both live in the same pond. You sampled 16 fry: 8 in the shallow water (2 were big and 6 were small); and 8 in deep water (2 were big and 6 were small). Size does not seem to be related to water depth. You recorded in your field notes that of the 16 fry sampled, 8 were caught in the vegetation (of which 2 were big and 6 were small); and 8 were caught in open water (of which 2 were big and 6 were small). Size does not seem to be related to vegetation.

You structure your fish sizes like this:

	Near vegetation	In open water	
Shallow water	5, 5	1, 1, 1, 1, 1, 1	16/8 = 2
Deep water	1, 1, 1, 1, 1, 1	5, 5	16/8 = 2
	16/8 = 2	16/8 = 2	32/16 = 2

The average size of all fish is $32/16 = 2$. The sum of squared error around 2 is:

$$4 \times 3 \times 3 + 12 \times 1 \times 1 = 48$$

The average size within each water depth is also 2 for each water depth. The sum of squared errors within the shallow water is:

$$2 \times 3 \times 3 + 6 \times 1 \times 1 = 24$$

The sum of squared errors within the deep water is:

$$6 \times 1 \times 1 + 2 \times 3 \times 3 = 24.$$

Total sum of squared errors after knowledge of within water depths is 24 + 24 = 48. Knowledge of water depth, a candidate for a cause, does not reduce squared error.

Calculate sum of squared error

Now apply this same analysis to the nearness to vegetation. Your result shows that knowledge of nearness to vegetation does not reduce sum of squared errors in fish size either. It seems that measuring water depth and nearness to vegetation has resulted in a negative result, in which what you have to report is that some of the causes that you measured do not explain some phenomenon of interest. Unfortunately, such negative results are not considered publishable by our western scientific community, unless some publications have already suggested that those causes might explain that phenomenon, i.e., you were testing some other scientist's hypothesis, and arguing to reject it, based on your data.

Two-way ANOVA

In any case, what you have done in reaching these conclusions is two one-way analyses of variance. You can combine these into one two-way analysis of variance with main effects using the linear model:

$$Y(i) = B0 + B1 \times X1(i) + B2 \times X2(i) + E(i)$$

X1 represents water depth: $X1(i) = -1$ if fish i is in shallow water and $X1(i) = +1$ if fish i is in deep water. X2 represents nearness to vegetation: $X2(i) = -1$ if fish i is near vegetation, $X2(i) = +1$ if fish i is in open water. $Y(i)$ is the size of fish i and $E(i)$ is the error in determining fish size i with this model. You use this linear model, called two-way analysis of variance in classical statistics, like this:

$$Y^T = (5\ 5\ 1\ 1\ 1\ 1\ 1\ 1\ 1\ 1\ 1\ 1\ 1\ 1\ 5\ 5)$$

The design matrix X for this linear model is:

$$X^T = \begin{pmatrix} 1 & 1 & 1 & 1 & 1 & 1 & 1 & 1 & 1 & 1 & 1 & 1 & 1 & 1 & 1 & 1 \\ -1 & -1 & -1 & -1 & -1 & -1 & -1 & -1 & 1 & 1 & 1 & 1 & 1 & 1 & 1 & 1 \\ -1 & -1 & 1 & 1 & 1 & 1 & 1 & 1 & -1 & -1 & -1 & -1 & -1 & -1 & 1 & 1 \end{pmatrix}$$

$$X^T \times X = \begin{pmatrix} 16 & 0 & 0 \\ 0 & 16 & -8 \\ 0 & -8 & 16 \end{pmatrix} \qquad C = 1/8 \times \begin{pmatrix} 1/2 & 0 & 0 \\ 0 & 2/3 & 1/3 \\ 0 & 1/3 & 2/3 \end{pmatrix}$$

$$X^T \times Y = \begin{pmatrix} 32 \\ 0 \\ 0 \end{pmatrix} \qquad C \times X^T \times Y = \begin{pmatrix} 2 \\ 0 \\ 0 \end{pmatrix} = \begin{pmatrix} B0 \\ B1 \\ B2 \end{pmatrix}$$

Thus, $Y(I) = 2 + 0 \times X1(I) + 0 \times X2(I) + E(I)$, which you already knew, but it is instructive to see the procedures work. You quietly approach your study pond one day and see wading shore birds. They catch and eat only big fry, unless of course they can't see them hidden in the vegetation. Quietly, you peer into the deeper water where big fry eat little fry, unless of course they can't see them hidden in the vegetation. In the ecosystem you are studying there is actually an interaction between water depth and nearness to vegetation, mediated by shore birds.

Interaction

Another linear model can represent this interaction:

$$Y[i] = B0 + B1 \times X1[i] \times X2[i] + E[i]$$

Check for yourself that:

$$X^T \times X = 8 \times \begin{pmatrix} 2 & -1 \\ -1 & 2 \end{pmatrix} \qquad C = 1/8 \times \begin{pmatrix} 2/3 & 1/3 \\ 1/3 & 2/3 \end{pmatrix}$$

$$X^T \times Y = \begin{pmatrix} 32 \\ 8 \end{pmatrix} \qquad C \times X^T \times Y = \begin{pmatrix} 3 \\ 2 \end{pmatrix}$$

Thus:

$$Y[i] = 3 + 2 \times X1[i] \times X2[i] + E[i]$$

Take a moment now to evaluate the errors. Considering both water depth and nearness to vegetation at the same time, you can see that variation in fish size can be completely explained in this way.

I contrived this example to resemble an ecological research project in which interactions play a dominant, in this case only, role in explaining how something of interest varies. Sometimes interactions have little importance. I have contrived for you another example to resemble an ecological research project in which two main effects contribute substantially to explaining variation.

No interaction

You count the number of flowers on eight *Impatiens capensis* plants that you find growing in a swale. Four of the plants are in sunnier spots and four are in less sunny spots; four of the plants are in wetter spots and four are in less wet spots. You structure the numbers of flowers on each plant like this:

	Number of flowers on plants in:		
	Sunnier spots	Less sunny spots	
Wetter spots	5, 5	3, 3	16/4 = 4
Not so wet spots	3, 3	1, 1	8/4 = 2
	16/4 = 4	8/4 = 2	24/8 = 3

Using 3 (the global mean) to represent the number of flowers gives a sum of squared error SSE0 = $4 \times 2 \times 2 + 4 \times 0 \times 0 = 16$. Using means within sunnier or less sunny spots gives a sum of squared errors, SSE1 = $4 \times 1 \times 1 + 4 \times 1 \times 1 = 8$. Thus knowledge of sunnier or less sunny reduces the SSE0 by 16 – 8 = 8; we say that it explains half the variance in number of flowers. Confirm that using means within wetter or not so wet spots gives a sum of squared error for wetness, SSE2 = 8, and so wetness also explains half the variation, but is it the other half? To find out, you can use the model:

$$Y[i] = B0 + B1 \times X1[i] + B2 \times X2[i] + E[i]$$

in which X1 represents sunnier vs less sunny, and X2 represents wetter vs not so wet. Arrange the eight Impatiens plants in the order in which they appear in the structure above, top row followed by the bottom row. Now, Y transpose looks like this:

$$Y^T = (5\ 5\ 3\ 3\ 3\ 3\ 1\ 1)$$

To make X, the design matrix, $X1(i) = 1$ if plant i grew in a sunnier spot, and $X1(i) = 0$ if plant i grew in a less sunny spot; similarly, $X2(i) = 1$ if plant i grew in a wetter spot, $X2(i) = 0$ if plant i grew in a less wet spot. Below, C has already been calculated by inverting X transpose X:

$$X^T = \begin{pmatrix} 1 & 1 & 1 & 1 & 1 & 1 & 1 & 1 \\ 1 & 1 & 0 & 0 & 1 & 1 & 0 & 0 \\ 1 & 1 & 1 & 1 & 0 & 0 & 0 & 0 \end{pmatrix} \quad C = 1/8 \times \begin{pmatrix} 3 & -2 & -2 \\ -2 & 4 & 0 \\ -2 & 0 & 4 \end{pmatrix}$$

Use important formula Equation 7.3 to confirm that B0 = 1, B1 = 2, and B2 = 2. Substitute these values for B0, B1, and B2, and use the linear model equation above to calculate the squared error. Did you get SSE = 0? From this you conclude that the two main effects each explain a separate half of the original error. In this case the main effects explain everything and the interaction explains nothing.

Re-coding

As an exercise, try re-coding X1 to equal –1 for plants in sunnier, and +1 for plants in less sunny, spots; and re-coding X2 to equal –1 for plants in wetter spots and +1 for plants in not so wet spots. Estimate the B0, B1, and B2 for this design matrix. If you do it right, you will have no trouble inverting X transpose X to get C. Does this model determine the same number of flowers under the same conditions? Does it explain the same squared error? (Hint: yes.)

You collected some more fish-size data a little later in the season when most of the birds had left. Now, the fish have grown a little and vary more continuously. These are your data:

	Near vegetation	In open water	
Shallow water	5, 6, 7	3, 4, 5	30/6 = 5
Deep water	1, 2, 3	7, 8, 9	30/6 = 5
	24/6 = 4	36/6 = 6	60/12 = 5

Use the same symmetric coding you used for Impatiens to make design matrices to model the main effects and their interaction separately, then to model the main effects together in a two-way model. All matrix inversions can be done by taking reciprocals of the main diagonal. Later in the season when the shore birds had migrated and the fish had grown bigger, did the interaction still completely explain fish size, or was there some variability left over to explain with main effects? How do the squared errors explained by the same effect differ among models?

Obviously, the creatures in these examples have been very co-operative so that you can see natural-looking cases of extreme interaction, and of no interaction. Considering wet and sun separately was sufficient to explain all the variance in flower number, so there is no more variance left to explain by an interaction between sun and wet. Of course even if there were variance left to explain, this would not mean that their interaction would explain it. The number of flowers might have nothing to do with either sun or wet or an interaction between sun and wet.

Combined linear model – A linear model can incorporate all three sources of possible explanation, the two main effects plus their interaction, to determine simultaneously their importance, like this:

$$Y(i) = B0 + B1 \times X1(i) + B2 \times X2(i) + B3 \times X1(i) \times X2(i) + E(i)$$

In this case, the design matrix has four columns, so you will need to invert a 4×4 matrix to determine C. Try this model with the Impatiens example using the second coding, as a sequel to the exercise that you have already done. You still should have no trouble inverting X transpose X to get C. In fact, you can use this design matrix for any data-gathering regime in which you have two effects, such as sun and wet, each of which distinguish two groups, and you measure the same number of things for each combination.

Use this same style of symmetric design matrix to make a simultaneous model of depth and vegetation to explain fish size using your late-season data. Here are some results to check your work: B0 = 5, B1 = 0, B2 = 1, B3 = 2, and SSE0 = 68. The water depth alone explains nothing. The vegetation alone explains 12. The interaction and the vegetation together explain 56. How much did the interaction alone explain? Eight out of 68 remain unexplained. Do the interaction and the vegetation explain some of the same variation?

Be reminded that these applications of the linear model serve to structure data, and partition variability among possible causes, using the criterion of minimizing squared error. No hypotheses of random variation have been considered and no test statistics have been explicitly described, although ideas from Section 7.4 can be applied. Fitting linear models, and using them to test hypotheses with data are separate tasks. You now have computational tools for approaching the latter task. If you have a balanced design, inverting X transpose X is a simple matter of taking reciprocals of the main diagonal.

Sub INVERSE

For unbalanced designs and for regression, I wrote a macro procedure to implement a simplified algorithm for matrix inversion that will work for design matrices of well-designed experiments (but not for all invertible matrices). It is shown below:

```
Sub INVERSE 'The calling sequence below should be on this line
    (N As Byte, OM() As Single, IM() As Single, FAIL As Boolean)
    'Finds inverse of OM, an N x N matrix, and puts it in IM
Dim I, J, R, C, MR As Byte
Dim DENO, SUBFAC As Single
Dim DONEROW(10) As Byte
Dim MAX As Single
FAIL = False
For R = 1 To N
    DONEROW(R) = 0    'no rows done yet
    Next R

For R = 1 To N
    For C = 1 To N
        If R = C Then
            IM(R, C) = 1.0
        Else
            IM(R, C) = 0.0   'put identity in IM
        End If
        Next C
    Next R
For J = 1 To N
    If Not FAIL Then
        MAX = 0.0
```

```
    For R = 1 To N          'Find row with biggest diagonal entry
    If DONEROW(R) = 0 Then
        If OM(R, R) >= MAX Then
            MAX = OM(R, R)
            MR = R
            End If 'If OM(R,
        If OM(R, R) + MAX <= 0# Then
            MAX = -OM(R, R)
            MR = R
            End If 'OM(R,
        End If 'DONEROW(R)
    Next R 'End For R = find row with biggest diagonal entry
DONEROW(MR) = 1
DENO = OM(MR, MR)
If (DENO > -0.001) And (DENO < 0.001) Then
    FAIL = True
    Else 'Divide row MR of each matrix by biggest diagonal
    'entry, subtract multiple from every other row
    For C = 1 To N ' divide
        OM(MR, C) = OM(MR, C) / DENO
        IM(MR, C) = IM(MR, C) / DENO
        Next C
    For R = 1 To N
        If R <> MR Then 'subtract
            SUBFAC = OM(R, MR) 'this is now 1 when R = MR
            For C = 1 To N
                OM(R, C) = OM(R, C) - OM(MR, C) * SUBFAC
                IM(R, C) = IM(R, C) - IM(MR, C) * SUBFAC
                Next C
            End If 'R <> MR
        Next R 'End For R
    End If 'End If (DENO >
End If 'Not FAIL

' For R = 1 To N 'Debug write
'       For C = 1 To N
'       Worksheets("Sheet1").Cells(R + 1 + J * (N + 1), C) = OM
        (R, C)
```

```
`       Next C
`       Next R
Next J 'End For J
End Sub 'Procedure INVERSE
```

Test Sub INVERSE

To test this procedure before trying to use it, and to show you how to use it in your own macros, I wrote the macro CALLINVERSE(). It reads the original matrix from the upper left corner of a spreadsheet, and writes its inverse beside it:

```
Sub CALLINVERSE()
Dim N As Byte
Dim ORIM(10, 10), INVM(10, 10) As Single
Dim FAIL As Boolean
Dim R, C As Integer
N = Worksheets("Sheet1").Cells(1, 1)
For R = 1 To N 'Read original matrix from Worksheet to test INVERSE
  For C = 1 To N
     ORIM(R, C) = Worksheets("Sheet1").Cells(R + 1, C)
     Next C
   Next R
Call INVERSE(N, ORIM(), INVM(), FAIL)
   If FAIL Then
     MsgBox ("INVERSE failed to invert this matrix")
     'End If
     Else
     MsgBox ("INVERSE inverted this matrix")
     End If 'End Else
   For R = 1 To N
     For C = 1 To N
        Worksheets("Sheet1").Cells(R + 1, C + N + 1) = INVM(R, C)
        Next C
     Next R
     End Sub
```

8 | Fitting distributions

8.1 Estimation of parameters

Estimators are random variables

You may choose to hypothesize variability using a random variable with a parametric distribution. Once you have hypothesized an appropriate family of parametric distributions, you still must hypothesize appropriate values for the parameters. If you have observed data, then one approach is to use your hypothesis that the observed data sampled a random variable with some distribution from that parametric family to estimate the parameters. This can be done in a variety of ways. Notice that your data are now assumed to be samples of a random variable. When you do arithmetic with the data to create an estimate of the parameters, such an estimate itself becomes a random variable, described by its distribution.

Hypothesize that your data have been generated by a binary random variable, **b**, repeatedly sampled independently, but you do not hypothesize a value for $p != \Pr(\mathbf{b} = 1)$. Instead you guess p from the data that you have observed. By what criteria could you make that guess? What properties might such guesses have?

Bias

Suppose you observe 1 1 0 0 1. You might estimate p with the guess, 0.6, using

x	$\Pr(\mathbf{pg} = x)$
.0/5	q^5
1/5	$5 \times p \times q^4$
2/5	$10 \times p^2 \times q^3$
3/5	$10 \times p^3 \times q^2$
4/5	$5 \times p^4 \times q$
5/5	p^5

the guessing rule **pg** != (**s5**)/5 where, as before, **s5** != **b**[1] + $\cdots$ + **b**[5]. Notice that this estimating formula defines another random variable based on the random variable hypothesized to have generated the observed data. The probability distribution of **pg** is binomial with $n = 5$. Denote as usual q != $1 - p$.

Calculate the expected value of this distribution like this:

$$E(\mathbf{pg}) = \sum_{i=0}^{5}(i/5 \times p^i \times q^{(5-i)} \times \text{binomial}[5, i])$$

$$E(\mathbf{pg}) = E((\mathbf{s5})/5) = E(\mathbf{s5})/5 = 5 \times E(\mathbf{b})/5 = E(\mathbf{b}) = p$$

This is very nice because the expected value of the random variable that we are using to estimate p is p itself. A random variable used for guessing the value of something that has an expected value equal to the value of the thing it is trying to guess is called unbiased. Otherwise it is called biased.

Accuracy

How good a guess does **pg** make? One way to evaluate an estimate is by its expected squared error, $E(\ (\mathbf{pg} - p)^2\ )$. The smaller the expected squared error, the better the guess it makes. For the same data, an estimator with a smaller expected squared error than another estimator is said to be more powerful. If a random variable for guessing is unbiased, then you can substitute its expected value for p above to see that its own variance measures its accuracy. The accuracy of the unbiased guessing random variable **pg** is:

$$\text{Var}(\mathbf{pg}) = \text{Var}((\mathbf{s5})/5) = \text{Var}(\mathbf{s5})/25 = 5 \times \text{Var}(\mathbf{b})/25 = \text{Var}(\mathbf{b})/5$$

Consistent

Suppose we had observed n samples. Now our guessing rule would be (**sn**)/n. The variance, $(p \times q)/n$, measures the accuracy of this guess. Thus, as we observe more data, the guess becomes more accurate. The limit as n becomes large of $E(((\mathbf{sn})/n - p)^2) = 0$. This means that if we could collect enough data then with high probability the guess will be as close as we want to p. Such a guessing rule is called consistent. An inconsistent estimator either gets close to the wrong thing, or it does not get close to anything, as more and more data are used.

Consider a weird estimator of p, **pwg** $!= (\mathbf{sn})/(n-1)$. This estimator is biased because its expected value is always bigger than p. But it is consistent because with enough data, its expected squared error can be as small as we want. Consider a very weird estimator of p, **pvwg** $!= (17 \times \mathbf{sn}/n - \mathbf{b}[1])/16$. This estimator is unbiased, but inconsistent; its expected squared error does not get close to zero no matter how many data are used.

Error as a random variable

Consider the linear model again. Hypothesize that observed bivariate data ($X(i)$ and $Y(i)$ observed for the same i) were generated by independent samples of a random variable, $\mathbf{e}$, with $\mathrm{Exp}(\mathbf{e}) = 0$. Sample $\mathbf{e}[i]$ determines the value of the ith response by the rule: $Y(i) = B0 + B1 \times X(i) + \mathbf{e}[i]$. You already know all the numbers $X(i)$ and $Y(i)$ because they are your design and observed responses. You have hypothesized that B0 and B1 are constant and invariant, but you do not know their values. You want to guess B0 and B1, based on the design $X(i)$ and the response $Y(i)$. To make the guesses B0g and B1g that minimize the squared error of the fit of your data to this linear model, you can call LINMO(N, X(), Y(), B0G, B1G, FAIL). Now the guesses **B0g** and **B1g** are random variables that result from arithmetic using samples of **e**.

Variance/covariance matrix

Without belaboring the matrix algebra, **B0g** and **B1g** are unbiased. This means $E(\mathbf{B0g}) = B0$ and $E(\mathbf{B1g}) = B1$. Because these estimators are unbiased, their accuracy is measured by their variances, $V(\mathbf{B0g})$ and $V(\mathbf{B1g})$. Their covariance, $\mathrm{CoV}(\mathbf{B0g},\mathbf{B1g})$, is related to the design, X. Consider again C $!= ((X^T \times X))^{-1}$, where X is the design matrix derived from the $X(i)$s. Without belaboring even more matrix algebra, we have:

$$\mathrm{Var}(\mathbf{B0g}) \quad = \mathrm{Var}(\mathbf{e}) \times C(1,1),$$
$$\mathrm{Var}(\mathbf{B1g}) \quad = \mathrm{Var}(\mathbf{e}) \times C(2,2) \text{ and}$$
$$\mathrm{CoV}(\mathbf{B0g},\mathbf{B1g}) = \mathrm{Var}(\mathbf{e}) \times C(1,2) = \mathrm{Var}(\mathbf{e}) \times C(2,1)$$

This is why C is called the variance/covariance matrix of the design.

The variability of the random variable, e, generates error. Even though the randomness comes from **e**, the errors in the estimates of B0 and B1 (their variances) are also affected by X, the design variables. An estimator is more accurate when its error is small. A design, X, with less error for the same amount of data is said to be more efficient. Covariance indicates redundancy in the design, which can be wasteful of efficiency. Especially in cases where it is expensive to collect data, consideration of efficient designs can be important. Look again at the linear model examples in Sections 7.3 and 7.4 Compare the variance/covariance matrices of the designs. The covariance (off diagonal) shows how efficient it is. A smaller covariance indicates a more efficient design. When the covariance is 0, the design has maximum efficiency.

Maximum likelihood

Consider another case of estimation. Variablers are well-known to be cross-eyed if they are dominant (XX or Xx) for the cross-eyed locus, else (xx) they are wall-eyed. An Xx parent has three offspring with a mate of unknown genotype. Assuming straightforward, Mendelian genetics, you can use the phenotypes of the offspring to guess the genotype of the mate with this table.

Number of cross-eyed offspring	Pr(mate is of given genotype)		
	XX	Xx	xx
0	0	$(1/4)^3 = 1/64$	$(1/2)^3 = 8/64$
1	0	$3 \times (1/4)^2 \times (3/4) = 9/64$	$3 \times (1/2)^{(2+2)} = 24/64$
2	0	$3 \times (1/4) \times (3/4)^2 = 27/64$	$3 \times (1/2)^{(2+2)} = 24/64$
3	1	$(3/4)^3 = 27/64$	$(1/2)^3 = 8/64$

For each of the four possible observations, 0, 1, 2, or 3 cross-eyed offspring, you can look across the row to see the conditional probabilities of making that observation, where the conditions are the possible unknown genotypes of the mate. Each column gives the conditional probability distribution for the sampled random variable, where the condition is the genotype at the top of the column. You could choose to guess the unknown genotype that made the sampled value of the random variable (number of cross-eyed offspring) most likely. A guessing rule with that property is called a maximum likelihood estimator. In this particular example, the estimator is a genotype-valued random variable, which cannot have an expected value or a variance because we cannot do the arithmetic with its values required in the definition of these concepts. So it cannot make sense to ask whether this estimator is biased or consistent or efficient, at least not in exactly the way those terms are defined.

This is how to find a maximum likelihood estimator for our first example, trying to guess $p = \Pr(\mathbf{b} = 1)$ based on n independent samples of $\mathbf{b}$. Consider again $\mathbf{sn} \mathrel{!=} \mathbf{b}[1] + \cdots + \mathbf{b}[n]$. Recall above that

$$\Pr(\mathbf{sn} = r) = p^r \times (1 - p)^{(n - r)} \times \text{binomial}[n, r].$$

What value of p will make this probability as large as possible? Note that the value of binomial$[n,r]$ does not change when p does, so we can choose the value, mp, that maximizes $mp^r \times (1 - mp)^{(n - r)}$. Call this %%%.

Logarithm is a monotone increasing function, so the same mp that maximizes %%% also maximizes Ln(%%%). Ln(%%%) is called the support function, S(mp). In this case, S(mp) = $r \times \text{Ln}(mp) + (n - r) \times \text{Ln}(1 - mp)$. To find the mp that makes S(mp) maximum, we take the derivative with respect to mp, and set it equal to zero, like this:

$$r/mp - (n - r)/(1 - mp) = 0$$

and solve for mp, to get $mp = r \mathbin{/} n$. Thus, the random variable $\mathbf{pg} = r \mathbin{/} n$ is unbiased, consistent, and maximum likelihood as an estimator of p.

Normal distribution

It is interesting to see what happens when we estimate the parameters of a normal distribution. We have n independent samples $\mathbf{x}[i]$ of a normally distributed random variable with expected value u and variance v, whose values we do not know. We want to use these n values of $\mathbf{x}[i]$ to estimate them. We can use the random variable $\mathbf{ug} \mathrel{=!} (\mathbf{x}[1] + \mathbf{x}[2] + .. + \mathbf{x}[n])/n$ to estimate u. You can easily confirm that Exp($\mathbf{ug}$) $= u$. Var($\mathbf{ug}$) $= v/n$, which gets closer to zero as you take more samples, so $\mathbf{ug}$ is consistent.

To discover the maximum-likelihood u-guessing random variable, call it $\mathbf{ugm}$, we need to use the normal distribution mathematical formula to write an expression for the likelihood of observing the $\mathbf{x}[i]$ values, when $\mathbf{ugm}$ has some particular value, call it mug. Then take its logarithm to get the support function. Without belaboring a lot of calculus, the derivative of the support function with respect to mug turns out to be:

$$\sum_{i=1}^{n} (x[i] - \text{mug})/v$$

which set to 0 can be solved for mug, the values of the parameter u (for a fixed v) that specify the normal distribution from which the n sampled values of $x[i]$ would have been most likely to have been observed. Is **ug** a maximum likelihood estimator of u? (Hint; yes.)

You can use a maximum likelihood approach to discover a maximum likelihood estimator **vgm** to guess variance, v. Without belaboring a lot more calculus, the derivative of the support function with respect to a value of **vgm** (call it mvg) turns out to be:

$$-n/(2 \times \text{mvg}) + \left(\sum_{i=1}^{n} ((x[i] - u)^2) \right)/(2 \times \text{mvg} \times \text{mvg})$$

which set to 0 gives

$$\text{mvg} = \left(\sum_{i=1}^{n} ((x[i] - u)^2) \right)/n$$

the average of the observed squared errors, a very intuitive result.

To appreciate further the parallel between our computational approach and formulas often encountered in classical statistics, let us consider again a normal distribution with expected value u and variance v, and as before the variance guessing random variable:

$$\text{vg} = !\left(\sum_{i=1}^{n} ((x[i] - u)^2) \right)/n$$

The question, What is the distribution of **vg**?, is interesting. One approach has been to standardize the normal distribution, square it and add n samples, like this:

$$\sum_{i=1}^{n} (((x[i] - u)/\text{SQRT}(v))^2)$$

Do you recognize that this has a Chi Square (CS) distribution with n degrees of freedom? Notice that:

$$v \times CS/n = \left(\sum_{i=1}^{n} \left((x[i] - u)^2 \right) \right) / n! = \mathbf{vg}$$

Thus, **vg** has a distribution proportional to Chi Square with n degrees of freedom.

Often we know neither the expected value nor the variance, so first we guess the expected value using **ug** and then use it to guess the variance, using:

$$\mathbf{vug} = !\left(\sum_{i=1}^{n} \left((x[i] - \mathbf{ug})^2 \right) \right) / n$$

Without belaboring the math, it turns out that if we use **ug** in the place of u, then Exp(**vug**) = $(n-1) \times v / n <> v$, i.e., **vug** is biased. To remove this bias, we can multiply **vg** by $n/(n-1)$ to get:

$$\mathbf{vwg}! = \left(\sum \left((x[i] - \mathbf{ug})^2 \right) \right) / (n-1)$$

which is the weird-guess, but unbiased estimator, which you may have seen as a formula.

Confidence interval

You can use **vg** or **vwg** to estimate a single value of v, but another approach is to determine a confidence interval for v. This is a range of values one of which is the true value of v with a given probability. The estimate **vwg** has the distribution $v/(n-1)$ times Chi Square with $n-1$ degrees, so $(n-1) \times \mathbf{vwg} / v$ is distributed as Chi Square with $n-1$ degrees. To determine a confidence interval using a classical approach, you need to consult a table of Chi Square distributions. But you can use computation to estimate the probability distribution for any well-defined random variable and so determine the reliability of estimators under its hypothesis.

Re-using data

Sometimes you use data to estimate a parameter of a parametric distribution that is part of a hypothesis from which you make predictions to compare with the same observed data. In such a case, you have deliberately chosen the member of the parametric family of distributions that best fits your data. This makes less convincing any argument that your data are consistent with your hypothesis, because you deliberately chose your hypothesis to be most consistent with your data. If the value of your test statistic is improbably high or low according to the distribution predicted by your hypothesis, then you argue that the aspect of your data measured by your test statistic is not consistent with your hypothesis. This argument is not less convincing, because even though you have chosen the hypothesis that best fits your data, they still do not fit very well. In Chapter 10, I will discuss in more detail the problem of peeking at your data to choose a hypothesis.

8.2 Goodness of fit

Test statistic

Hypothesize that n observations independently sample the binary random variable, **b**, with distribution $\Pr(\mathbf{b} = 1) = p$. You want to use these observations to test your hypothesis. By analogy, your hypothesis states that the mechanism that produced your observations did so as if independently sampling the random variable **b**. To test your hypothesis you need a test statistic. One commonly used for this purpose by classical statistics is calculated using two new random variables: **sn1** != the number of times you observe **b** = 1; and **sn0** != the number of times you observe **b** = 0. Because **sn0** + **sn1** = n, **sn1** and **sn0** are NOT independent random variables. The classical statistic is calculated from a sample of **sn1**[1] like this:

$$CS[1] \; ! = \frac{(sn1[1] - n \times p)^2}{n \times p} + \frac{(sn0[1] - n \times (1 - p))^2}{n \times (1 - p)}$$

From Chapter 4 you know that $E(\mathbf{sn1}) = n \times p$ and $E(\mathbf{sn0}) = n \times (1-p)$.

There are two groups of observations: **b** = 1 or **b** = 0. For each group, you subtract the number expected from the number observed and then divide the square of this difference by the number expected; finally you add these two quotients. If you observe numbers close to those you expect, then **CS**[1] will be small and you will argue that the observations are consistent with your hypothesis. If you observe numbers far from those you expect, then **CS**[1] will be big and you will argue that your observations contradict your hypothesis. To determine what values for **CS**[1] should be interpreted as big or small you need to know the probability distribution for the random variable **CS** predicted by your hypothesis.

By now, you know how to compute an accurate estimate of the probability distribution predicted by your hypothesis for the test statistic **CS**[1]. It might be useful for you to write a macro to do it. Of course, if you take a computational approach, you would not need to define such a complicated test statistic: **sn1**[1]− $n \times p$, or even **sn1**[1] itself, would have been adequate. However, the test statistic **CS**[1] is used in classical statistics because the distribution predicted for it by the hypothesis in question here asymptotically converges, as n gets large, to the pre-calculated distribution called Chi Square. Its percentiles are published in the backs of statistics books, and even stored in computers so that programs that calculate classical statistics can look them up there.

Derive Chi Square

As you have now seen, the Chi Square distribution is central to many applications in classical statistics, and related concepts are applicable to tests of hypotheses to explain the natural world. Thus, I will discuss Chi Square in more detail, which will show you how the Chi Square distribution originates in the simple case above. The results generalize to the more general case, but the arguments to demonstrate this are beyond the scope of this book. To simplify notation, I will write the sample, **sn1**[1], simply as **sn1**.

Start by rewriting **sn1** − $n \times p$ in a sequence of equivalent ways.

$$\textbf{sn1} - n \times p = \textbf{sn1} + 0 - n \times p \quad \text{add 0, substitute}$$
$$= (n - \textbf{sn0}) + n \times (1 - p) - n \times (1 - p) - n \times p$$
$$\text{fancy name for 0}$$
$$= -\textbf{sn0} + n \times (1 - p) + n - n \times ((1 - p) + p)$$
$$\text{re-arrange ()}$$
$$= -\textbf{sn0} + n \times (1 - p) \quad \text{cancel } n, \text{ and}$$
$$-(\textbf{sn1} - n \times p) = \textbf{sn0} - n \times (1 - p) \quad \text{change signs.}$$

Now, substitute this into the above expression for **CS**:

$$CS = \frac{(\text{sn1} - n \times p)^2}{n \times p} + \frac{(-(\text{sn1} - n \times p))^2}{n \times (1 - p)}$$

Combine over the common denominator, $n \times p \times (1 - p)$:

$$CS = \frac{(\mathbf{sn1} - n \times p)^2 \times (1 - p) + (\mathbf{sn1} - n \times p)^2 \times p}{n \times p \times (1 - p)}$$

Now, finally add together the terms of the numerator to get:

$$CS! = \frac{(\mathbf{sn1} - n \times p)^2}{n \times p \times (1 - p)}$$

Thus, **CS** is the square of a standardized binomial. As n gets large, a standardized binomial gets close to a normal distribution with expected value zero and variance 1. So as n gets larger, the distribution of **CS** approximates more and more closely the square of a standardized normal distribution, which we call the Chi Square distribution.

Use Chi Square

One common use of Chi Square is a generalization of the hypothesis testing discussed above. It tests the hypothesis that a particular group of samples comes from a specified distribution. This test is called goodness of fit. Suppose there are n independent samples $\mathbf{x}[1], \mathbf{x}[2], .., \mathbf{x}[n]$ of a random variable $\mathbf{x}$ with an unknown distribution. Is this group of n samples consistent with the hypothesis that they were taken from a specified, known distribution? One way to answer this question is to divide the samples into two groups by putting in one group samples with values $\leq t$ and in the other group samples with values $> t$. Under this hypothesis, the probability that a sample $\mathbf{x}[j]$ has a value in the first group is $\Pr(\mathbf{x}[j] \leq t) != p$. The value of p is known because the distribution specified by the hypothesis is known. Denote with $\mathbf{sn1}[1]$ the observed number of samples $\leq t$, and with $\mathbf{sn0}[1]$ the observed number of samples $>t$. Now you compute the observed value for $\mathbf{CS}[1]$ and look up its realized significance in the Chi Square table in a statistics book.

This compares the hypothesized distribution only with the probabilities of drawing a sample either side of the threshold, t. The distribution of your sample values within either one of these two intervals might differ wildly from your hypothesized distribution. To create a test statistic that measures more closely how well your samples fit your hypothesized distribution, you can divide your samples into m groups by specifying $m - 1$ thresholds. You know the probabilities, $p1, p2, .. pm$, that sample $x[j]$ has a value in interval i because you know the distribution specified by your hypothesis. With n samples, the expected number of samples with values in interval i would be $pi \times n$. Calculate the observed statistic; the sum over all m groups of (the squared deviation of the observed from the expected) divided by the expected. Using manipulations analogous to those above, which I will not belabor, this statistic can be shown to have a distribution that approximates the sum of $m - 1$ squared independent samples of a standardized normal distribution, called Chi Square with $m - 1$ degrees of freedom. In the original example above, there was only one threshold making two groups ($m = 2$), and an approximation to a standard normal distribution was sampled only once to calculate a value for the test statistic. This statistic has a distribution that approximates Chi Square with $m - 1 = 1$ degree of freedom. Because the number n of samples of x is fixed, after you count the number of samples with values in the first $m - 1$ intervals, the number with values in interval m is already known, so it is not free to vary. The Chi Square distribution is different for each number of degrees of freedom, so Chi Square is a family of parametric distributions with degrees of freedom as its parameter. For each value of degrees of freedom up to well over 100, percentiles of the corresponding Chi Square distribution have been calculated and published in tables.

Accuracy of Chi Square

To test whether samples of an unknown random variable x could be plausibly construed to be sampling a given distribution, you can divide the range into m intervals and calculate the statistic above whose distribution is approximately Chi Square with $m - 1$ degrees of freedom. To approximate the Chi Square distribution with convincing accuracy, $n \times \Pr(x[j]$ is in interval i), which is the expected number of samples with values in interval i, should be large for every interval. If for some interval, the expected number of observations is less than five, the approximation to the normal distribution for that interval is generally considered so poor that the distribution of the test statistic **CS** does not approximate the Chi Square distribution very well. This presents a trade-off: for a given number n of samples, the more intervals (bigger m) the more closely the counts of samples in the m intervals can track the shape of the distribution that you hypothesized, but for at least some intervals their expected number of sample values will be lower. Thus for fixed n, more intervals lowers the accuracy with which the distribution of **CS** approximates Chi Square.

Calculate the predicted distribution

You can now use computational techniques to create your own good estimate of distributions of test statistics that measure goodness of fit by sampling the known distribution as many times as you have samples of **x**, the unknown random variable, and calculating the value of the test statistic. By repeating this 1000 (or more) times you get an accurate estimate of the predicted distribution of the test statistic that measures goodness of fit. One relevant test statistic to measure goodness of fit is **CS**, discussed above. Using a computational approach, you can estimate the realized significance of an observed value **CS**[1] more accurately than by using the Chi Square distribution. With small expected values of number of samples in the m intervals, a computational estimate of the realized significance of **CS**[1] is more accurate. In calculating a value for **CS**, the squared differences between observed and expected are scaled in units of the expected value for their interval, which reduces the contribution of intervals with larger expected values and increases the contribution of intervals with smaller expected values. Whether or not this is most appropriate to what you want to measure, **CS** has to do it this way so that its predicted distribution will asymptotically approach Chi Square as n gets larger. With a computational approach, you can use any statistic that you can calculate. Another relevant statistic to test goodness of fit is the sum over m intervals of the squared differences between observed number of sample values and their expected number. This does not scale the contribution of each interval by its expected value. Another relevant statistic to test goodness of fit is the sum over m intervals of absolute difference between observed number of sample values and their expected number. This does not give big differences relatively more weight than small differences. Another statistic is to take each sample value in turn, calculate the expected number of samples greater than or equal to that value and compare it to the observed number of samples using the absolute difference; the maximum of these absolute differences is the value of the statistic.

Even though with calculation your choice of statistic is liberated and the distribution predicted for that statistic can be estimated accurately, the power to reject a false hypothesis still increases with increasing number n of observations. Thus, if you have only a few observations (small n) they are likely to be consistent with a wide variety of hypothesized distributions, no matter how creatively or accurately you test them.

Iberian demography

Recall the example of Chapter 1, in which age at death for a small sample of males in a rural village in Portugal surviving childhood and dying near the end of the nineteenth century, is compared with two different distributions: age at death in rural Spain and age at death in urban Portugal, both estimated near the same time. One approach to this question is goodness of fit. Do the samples from rural Portugal seem more as if drawn from the distribution of rural Spain or more as if drawn from the distribution of urban Portugal? With only 14 samples, it would probably be good to divide the ages at death in rural Portugal into just three intervals: approximately the youngest third, the oldest third, and the middle third. You could use as the test statistics the numbers of males in the rural Portuguese village observed to have died in each age interval. Then sample the age at death distribution for rural Spain 14 times to simulate the rural Portuguese observations. Compare simulated numbers in each of the three age classes to observed, and increment significance counters. Do this 1000 times to estimate realized significances for observed counts. You would do the same, sampling the age at death for urban Portugal. Of course with so few observations, it would not be surprising if you failed to reject either hypothesis; but not because the distributions predicted for your test statistics were not accurate. With so few samples, they could seem like samples of either distribution.

9 | Dependencies

9.1 Interpreting mixtures

Sometimes the data that you observe seem to have been produced by a mixture of different random processes. Here I present examples of data that have been produced by two random processes mixed in two different ways. Using these examples, I show you how to test a hypothesis to determine whether data seem to be the result of two different random processes, mixed in one of these two different ways.

Variablers

Common Variablers typically lay two eggs in their nest. The two chicks can be both male, one male and one female, or both female. Denote with p the probability that a chick is male. Thus, the number of males in any particular nest is a random variable, X, with distribution:

$$Pr(X = 2) = p \times p$$
$$Pr(X = 1) = 2 \times p \times (1 - p)$$
$$Pr(X = 0) = (1 - p) \times (1 - p)$$

This distribution for X (the number of males) is predicted by the hypothesis that p is the same for all chicks in all nests. Recall that the expected value for X is given by $E(X) = 2 \times p$, and that the variance of X is given by $V(X) = 2 \times p \times (1 - p)$.

Greater Variablers also lay two eggs per nest, but for half the mated pairs the probability that a chick is male is $p + m$. For the other half the probability that a chick is male is $p - m$.

The distribution of **X** for Greater Variablers is:

$$\Pr(\mathbf{X} = 2) = 1/2 \times (p + m)^2 + 1/2 \times (p - m)^2$$
$$= p^2 + m^2$$
$$\Pr(\mathbf{X} = 1) = 2/2 \times (p + m) \times (1 - (p+m)) + 2/2 \times (p - m) \times (1 - (p - m))$$
$$= 2 \times p \times (1 - p) - 2 \times m^2$$
$$\Pr(\mathbf{X} = 0) = 1/2 \times (1 - (p + m))^2 + 1/2 \times (1 - (p - m))^2$$
$$= (1 - p)^2 + m^2$$

Note that among Greater Variablers, if you do not know from which half the parents come, then the probability is still p that a chick is male. Check the arithmetic to confirm that:

$$E(\mathbf{X}) = 2 \times p \text{ and } Var(\mathbf{X}) = 2 \times p \times (1 - p) + 2 \times m \times m$$

Among Lesser Variablers, the first egg laid is more likely to be male with probability $p + m$ and the second egg is less likely to be male with probability $p - m$, but this is the same for all pairs of parental birds. Shown below is the distribution of **X** (the number of males in a nest) in Lesser Variablers:

$$\Pr(\mathbf{X} = 2) = (p + m) \times (p - m)$$
$$= p^2 - m^2$$
$$\Pr(\mathbf{X} = 1) = (1 - (p + m)) \times (p - m) + (p + m) \times (1 - (p - m))$$
$$= 2 \times p \times (1 - p) + 2 \times m^2$$
$$\Pr(\mathbf{X} = 0) = (1 - (p + m)) \times (1 - (p - m)) = (1 - p) - m^2$$

Note that for Lesser Variablers, if you do not know which egg was laid first, then the probability is still p that a chick is male. Check the arithmetic to confirm that:

$$E(\mathbf{X}) = 2 \times p \text{ and } V(\mathbf{X}) = 2 \times p \times (1 - p) - 2 \times m \times m$$

As you have seen, the expected number of males is the same for all Variablers, but the variance in the number of males is greater for Greater Variablers and less for Lesser Variablers.

It is extremely difficult to tell Lesser Variablers from Greater Variablers by observing their morphology or behavior, but people who grind them up and put them through a DNA machine assure us that they are really quite different. But you do not need their DNA because you can tell them apart by their variance!

Statistically savvy scientists who study Variablers always hypothesize that they are Common Variablers. They use an estimate of the variance as their test statistic. They predict a probability distribution for their estimate of variance. They compare their variance estimate to its predicted distribution to determine its realized significance under the Common Variabler hypothesis. If the estimate of variance is improbably high then they conclude that they are studying Greater Variablers; if it is improbably low then they conclude that they are studying Lesser Variablers.

Actually, no one has ever seen a Common Variabler, and scientists are beginning to suspect that they never existed, or have gone extinct a long time ago. But they continue to hypothesize that they are studying them, because they can use the predictions that this hypothesis makes to interpret data to tell whether they have observed Greater or Lesser Variablers, or their very common conceptual equivalents.

Use the null hypothesis

The null Common Variabler hypothesis is the parametric family of binomial distributions for **s2**, with $n = 2$ and p the parameter. You study a population of Variablers by observing a large number, n, of nests and for each you record the number of male chicks: 0, 1, or 2. To test whether these numbers are consistent with the Common Variabler hypothesis that the probability p that any egg hatch into a male chick is the same for all eggs, you construe each observed nest as a sample of the random variable **X**. To determine a distribution for **X** you need to know the value of p. Because you cannot observe p directly, you make an estimate **pg**[1] (i.e., p-guess) of p like this: **pg**[1] != (number of males observed)/($2 \times$ number of nests observed).

Supposed you observed the nests of a number (POV) of Pairs Of Variablers and put the estimate **pg**[1] in place PG. You can write macro statements to use the Common Variabler hypothesis to generate a data set with POV nests, and determine the Number Of Males, NOM(), in each nest, NEST, as shown above:

```
For NEST = 1 To POV
    NOM(NEST) = 0
    If Rnd < PG Then
        NOM(NEST) = NOM(NEST) + 1;
    End If
    If Rnd < PG Then
        NOM(NEST) = NOM(NEST) + 1;
    End If
    Next NEST
```

Effect of test statistic on your argument

One test statistic relevant to the question might be an estimate of the variance of X using the deviations from $2 \times p$ of observed numbers of males in each nest. But you cannot calculate this because you do not actually know the value of p. So you might settle for a not quite so convincing test statistic, $\mathbf{vg}[1]$ (i.e., V-guess) based on the value $\mathbf{pg}[1]$ that you estimated for p:

$$\mathbf{vg}[1]! = \sum_{i=1}^{POV} (2 \times \mathbf{pg}[1] - \mathbf{X}[i])2/POV$$

To estimate a predicted distribution for $\mathbf{vg}[1]$, you use the Common Variabler hypothesis to simulate 1000 (say) data sets and use each to calculate a value for $\mathbf{vg}$. This raises an interesting question: do you estimate the variance of X with the simulated data set using $\mathbf{pg}[1]$, or do you first calculate $\mathbf{spg}[i]$ (an estimate of p using the ith simulated data set) and use that to estimate the variance of X for the ith simulated data set? Note that using $\mathbf{spg}[i]$ calculates the average squared error around the mean of the simulated data. Recall that the mean is the value that minimized squared error. Thus, except in rare cases where $\mathbf{pg}[1] = \mathbf{spg}[i]$, using $\mathbf{pg}[1]$ will result in larger simulated values for the test statistic, which will tend to make the observed value of the test statistic appear smaller in the context of the distribution predicted for it by the Common Variabler hypothesis.

Often, the most effective choice depends on what you want to argue. In general, if you can make choices of this kind that are hostile to the interpretation that you want to argue, but still have statistical support for your argument, your argument is more convincing. In this case, if you wanted to argue that you were actually studying Lesser Variablers, choosing **spg**[1] will produce a predicted distribution for the test statistic that will make it harder to reject Common Variablers in favor of Lesser Variablers. If you still had statistical support for Lesser Variablers, your argument would be stronger than if you had chosen **pg**[1].

Catalpa speciosa

You have recognized by now that the Variablers are an artificial example that I invented to illustrate some of the concepts involved. However, there are many natural situations where these concepts are relevant. For example, *Catalpa speciosa* (the Indiana banana) is a tree in the little-known plant family Bignoniaceae. It reaches its northern limit near the University of Michigan. There, it flowers on the summer solstice, presenting a huge display of white flowers tinged with pink. The display is so attractive it is planted on the streets of Ann Arbor.

Catalpa speciosa is unusual in that it makes three leaves at a node, and thus initiates three branches from the three axils there. Usually only one branch grows, so the branching pattern ends up looking ordinary. When the branch tips bear inflorescences they branch three times in threes to produce 27 flowers. They are bee pollinated by day and moth pollinated by night. During the day, *Catalpa speciosa* makes concentrated nectar to please the bees, but at night it makes dilute nectar to please the moths, who need to suck it up through their long, very thin proboscises. With its huge floral display and circadian nectar, these qualities of *Catalpa speciosa* appear to be the result of natural selection to increase the chances that its flowers will get pollinated. After a frenzy of pollination activity night and day for a short week around midsummer's night, *Catalpa speciosa* drops its thousands of flowers onto the ground, and begins to develop fruits.

You collect 10 *Catalpa speciosa* branch tips and count the number of fruits beginning to develop. These are your numbers:

$$3 \quad 5 \quad 4 \quad 0 \quad 3 \quad 1 \quad 3 \quad 4 \quad 1 \quad 3$$

You wonder: does each flower have the same chance of becoming a fruit OR do some inflorescences have a higher probability of turning their flowers into fruits than others OR do some flowers within an inflorescence have a higher probability of becoming fruits than others in the same inflorescence? You can see how understanding Variablers helps you answer this question. Make a hypothesis, choose a test statistic, and write a macro to estimate a predicted probability distribution to help you argue which of these explanations seems most credible.

9.2   Series of dependent random variables

Dependency

There are several reasons why it is useful to hypothesize independence. If we cannot reject independence, then descriptions of how things depend on one another may not be justified. Often, the way that a hypothesis of independence is rejected suggests a possible mechanism of dependence, as with Variablers. Independence is usually a simpler concept with a limited number of reasonable mechanisms to implement it, but there are usually a large number of different ways that things could depend one another, and the more dimensions of complexity you use, the easier it is to explain things and so the less convincing becomes the explanation. This is especially so when you use your observed data to estimate parameters for several dimensions of explanatory complexity. This is why it is nice to have alternatives to independence that hypothesize simple enough mechanisms that our observations can still fail to fit, if they are in fact inconsistent.

Random walk

Consider the binary random variable $\mathbf{b}$ with distribution $\Pr(\mathbf{b} = 1) = p$, $\Pr(\mathbf{b} = -1) = (1 - p)$. Define a series $\mathbf{w1}, \mathbf{w2}, .. \mathbf{wi}, \mathbf{wj} ..$ of random variables with $\mathbf{w1} \mathrel{!=} \mathbf{b}$ and $\mathbf{wj} \mathrel{!=} \mathbf{wi} + \mathbf{b}$ where $j \mathrel{!=} i + 1$. For example, $\mathbf{w3}$ has a distribution, but if we know the value of $\mathbf{w2}$ this knowledge changes the distribution of $\mathbf{w3}$. Highly stylized dependencies of this kind are called random walks. Where you are next depends in part on where you are now. A random walk is a particular kind of auto-regressive series.

Auto-regressive series

The concept of random walk can be generalized with time (or space) series called auto-regressive. Suppose that $\mathbf{X1}, \mathbf{X2}, \ldots$ is a series of random variables sampled at regular time intervals: $X1[1]$ at time 1, $X2[2]$ at time 2, etc. They might be independent and identically distributed. These properties are so commonly assumed that we denote them, iid. But they might be related by the formula $Xt = B0 + B1 \times Xs + e$ in which $s = t - 1$ and e is a single random variable whose distribution does not vary with time, i.e., e is stationary. You could estimate B0 and B1 by doing a least-squares regression, with the Ys equal to the observed Xs displaced by one time unit. If B0 were 0 and B1 were 1, then you would have a random walk in which each step (time unit) was a sample of e. If B1 were 0, then the Xs would be independent samples of e (plus the constant B0). If the value of B1 is different from 0, then we call the Xs an AR1 series (Auto Regressive with 1 time unit). Sometimes there are dependencies that go back two time units. To look for them, fit:

$$Xt = B0 + B1 \times Xs + B2 \times Xr + e \text{ where } r = s - 1$$

If B2 is different from 0, then this is an AR2 series.

Markov process

Sometimes, a series of random variables all share the same small range of possible values, and their probabilities depend on the value of the random variable previously sampled. In such cases the values are often qualitative and are called states. For example, suppose that there are two alleles R and D at a locus; diploid organisms can exist in one of three states: DD, DR, or RR. In a breeding program, progeny are successively bred to a mate of genotype DR. Assuming no genetic subtleties, this could be described with a matrix of conditional probabilities, in which the rows represent the genotype of a parent and the columns represent the genotype of a child. The rows are conditional probability distributions for the possible genotypes of the child, given the genotype of the parent.

		Genotype of child after mating with DR		
		DD	DR	RR
Genotype or parent	DD	1/2	1/2	0
	DR	1/4	1/2	1/4
	RR	0	1/2	1/2

The entire matrix, P, is called a transition matrix. The series of genotypes of successive generations of children is defined by the matrix, P. A series that can be defined in this way is called a Markov process or a Markov Chain. A Markov process is said to be ergodic if it can eventually get from any state to any other state; it is called regular (a special case of ergodic) if it can get from any state to any other state in exactly the same number of steps.

Suppose a Markov process starts in some state, goes through two transitions, to end up in some state. The conditional probability distributions giving the probabilities for where it will end up are the rows in the matrix $P \times P$, in which $\times$ is ordinary matrix multiplication. Now that is pretty remarkable, but if you try a couple of examples you will see that it works. If a regular Markov process goes on for a while, say n transitions, the transition matrix P^n gets close to a matrix T in which the rows are all equal (if w is the first row, the w is also the second row, etc.). The Markov process forgot where it started. In fact, $w \times P = w$, so we can use this to solve for w to discover the long-term, limiting probability distribution. Consult the celebrated text, Kemeny (1964), to learn more about Markov chains.

Test for a Markov process

How could you test a hypothesis that a series of observations through time could be explained as a Markov process? First, it would be a good idea to show that it could not be credibly explained by a simpler mechanism, such as independent, identically distributed, (iid) random variables. You could hypothesize iid, the probability with which each state is observed is the same for all times, and proportional to the frequency of that state in the entire observed series. You could then use this hypothesis to simulate a thousand series, each as long as the observed series. Now you need a test statistic, TS, to measure something about what you intend to test for. You then evaluate TS for the observed series, and for each of the simulated series, to count the number of simulated series for which the simulated value of TS is $\leq$ (and for which its value is $\geq$) the value of TS for the observed series.

To choose such a test statistic, consider the table below for a time series with possible states A, B, and C, in which the entries are the number of times in an observed series that the column state follows the row state:

		State following			
		A	B	C	
State	A	10	5	3	18
	B	5	4	3	12
preceding	C	3	3	0	6
		18	12	6	

In this example series, 37 states were observed. State A followed some state 18 out of 36 times, state B followed some state 12 out of 36 times, and state C followed some state 6 out of 36 times. Under an iid hypothesis, we could estimate the probability of observing A to be 1/2, B to be 1/3, and C to be 1/6, all proportional to their frequency of being unconditionally observed to follow some state. The probabilities of preceding something could be estimated in the same way. In this particular example the row and column frequencies turn out to be the same. The numbers expected in the matrix would be the probability of coming before times the probability of coming after times 36 observations of each kind. For example, the expected number of times that B would follow A would be $1/2 \times 1/3 \times 36 = 6$, but the observed number of times was only 5, which is a discrepancy of 1. Let the test statistic, TS, be the sum over all nine boxes of the absolute values of these discrepancies. If TS is too big, as indicated by the realized significances estimated by simulation, the observed series does not seem to be consistent with iid, but if TS is not too big, then the series (at least the sum of its discrepancies) is consistent with iid.

Notice that the iid hypothesis AND the test statistic work together to make a convincing argument in this case. There are many ways in which a series could fail to be iid. The test statistic measures one particular way, deliberately chosen to indicate a Markov process as an alternative. If the series were iid, then the rows in the count matrix represent three conditional frequency distributions that should be proportional to their marginal distribution; if the time series were generated by a Markov process, then the rows would not be expected to be proportional to the margin. However, there are many ways in which a series could fail to be iid, some still producing rows proportional to their margin. The example matrix above was derived from a series generated by sampling (A, B, C) independently 18 times with probability distribution (1/3, 1/3, 1/3), and then sampling 18 more times with probability distribution (2/3, 1/3, 0). This is not a Markov process, but neither is it iid. The test statistic, TS, has a realized significance under iid of about 0.7. TS is looking for a series, like a Markov process, that does not give rows of the transition matrix proportional to the margin. In this example, each observation is independent of its previous one, but the probability distribution is not stationary.

Keep in mind that estimating a Markov process involves hypothesizing several conditional probability distributions. If you use observed frequencies in the data to estimate all these numbers, it is not surprising that this will describe a Markov process that fits the observed data quite well in most cases. If you have a long enough series, sometimes it is convincing to use some of it to estimate conditional probability distributions, and the rest of it to test the predictions of the Markov process whose conditional probability distributions were estimated.

Absorbing Markov process

In contrast to fitting a Markov process to observed data, sometimes the concept is useful for describing simple dependencies in a context where you are attempting to understand other questions. One kind of NON-ergodic Markov chain that is of interest is the so-called absorbing Markov process. Suppose E(t) is a series of observations generated by a Markov process in which the probability is 1.0 that E(t) = A given that E(t - 1) = A . In such a Markov process, A is called an absorbing state, because once the process enters state A it gets stuck there; we say that it is absorbed in state A. A Markov process is called an absorbing Markov process if it has at least one absorbing state, and it is possible to get from any state to an absorbing state.

An absorbing Markov process will eventually get stuck in an absorbing state. Some interesting questions to ask about an absorbing Markov process include:

(1) With what probability will the process get stuck in any particular absorbing state?
(2) How long will it take on average for the process to get stuck?
(3) How many times on average will the process be in any of the non-absorbing states before it get stuck?

Consider, for example, a simplified model of succession on a plot of recently abandoned farm land that had been cleared 100 years ago by cutting down an Oak–Hickory forest. Suppose that on any given spot one of four kinds of plants can grow: *Centaurea, Daucus, Carya or Quercus* (i.e., Bachelor's Button, Queen Ann's Lace, Hickory, or Oak). Once an Oak or a Hickory establishes in a spot it stays there. If there is a Bachelor's Button one year, half the time it will still be there the next year, but it might be replaced by a Queen Ann's Lace, or possibly an Oak. If there is a Queen Ann's Lace about half the time it will be replaced next year by a Bachelor's Button, but it could remain Queen Ann's Lace or be replaced by a Hickory. From one year to the next we have this transition matrix, T:

		This year			
		o	b	q	h
Last year	o	1	0	0	0
	b	1/6	1/2	1/3	0
	q	0	1/2	1/3	1/6
	h	0	0	0	1

You can see that T is an absorbing Markov chain with two absorbing states, Oak and Hickory. In this context the questions become:

(1) What are the expected proportions of Oaks and Hickories in the climax forest?
(2) On average, how long will it take for a tree to establish?
(3) What will be the mix of Bachelor's Button and Queen Ann's Lace during succession?

The answers to these questions depend of the starting state of any particular place, so they will have the form of little matrices. Start by re-arranging T so that the absorbing states are first:

	o	h	b	q			
o	1	0	0	0			
h	0	1	0	0	!=	I	O
b	1/6	0	1/2	1/3		R	Q
q	0	1/6	1/2	1/3			

The transition matrix T is made up of four little matrices:

I = an identity matrix
O = a matrix of all zeros
R = get absorbed next
Q = do not get absorbed

The entries of the matrix N, with rows and columns: Bachelor's Button and Queen Ann's Lace, are defined to be the average number of times a place in the vegetation is in state column given that it started in state row. To discover N, start in a row and enact the process. It is in the column state already (I), plus if not absorbed it goes there next (Q), plus if still not absorbed it goes there after that (Q×Q), etc.

Thus, $N = I + Q + Q \times Q + Q \times Q \times Q + \cdots$

LOOK! $I + Q + Q \times Q + \cdots$
× $I - Q$

$$\begin{array}{l} I + Q + Q \times Q + Q \times Q \times Q \cdots \\ - Q - Q \times Q - Q \times Q \times Q \cdots \end{array}$$

=   I

Evidently, $N = (I - Q)^{-1}$

$$N = \begin{pmatrix} 1 - 1/2 & -1/3 \\ -1/2 & 1 - 1/3 \end{pmatrix}^{-1}$$

$N =$

	b	q
b	4	2
q	3	3

A place that has now Bachelor's Button will have a Bachelor's Button four times (on average) and have a Queen Ann's Lace two times (on average) before growing a tree. A place that has now a Queen Ann's Lace will have a Queen Ann's Lace three times (on average) and have a Bachelor's Button three times (on average) before growing a tree.

Notice that the sum of the rows of N is the answer to question 2. Denote with the matrix B the answer to question 1. The rows of B are the non-absorbing states and the columns of B are the absorbing states. Notice that a place is either absorbed on the next step or it becomes a non-absorbing state and then gets absorbed eventually from there. Saying this in matrices, $B = R + Q \times B$. Remember, B gives the probability that the process will be absorbed from wherever it went with the probabilities in Q. Re-arranging the above gives $B - Q \times B = R$. Factoring out B gives $(I - Q) \times B = R$. Multiplying on the left by $(I - Q)^{-1} = N$ gives $B = N \times R$.

In the case of the example, solving for B gives

	o	h
b	2/3	1/3
q	1/2	1/2

So if the whole field started as Bachelor's Button, you would expect 2/3 of the climax forest to be Oaks and 1/3 to be hickories, but if the whole field started as Queen Ann's Lace, half of the climax forest would be Oaks and half hickories. Other starting mixtures would give intermediate climax mixtures.

Example problem – Test your understanding with the following exercise. On any given day Spororks hide (H), eat (E), have been killed by a visual predator (V), or have been killed by an olfactory predator (O). If they hide today, then by tomorrow they have been killed by an olfactory predator with probability 1/5, hide again tomorrow with probability 1/10, and eat tomorrow with probability 7/10. If they eat today, then by tomorrow they have been killed by a visual predator with probability 2/5, hide tomorrow with probability 1/5, and eat again tomorrow with probability 2/5. If a Sporork is hiding today, with what probability will it be killed eventually by V? By O? How long on average will it live? If a Sporork is eating today, answer the same questions. Hints to solve this: set up the transition matrix and notice the absorbing states. Recognize the four little matrices. Do the matrix algebra. See the analogies and answer the questions about Sporork demography.

Describe spatial distribution

Estabrook and Jespersen (1974) used a Markov process to describe how two different kinds of prey species might be distributed in two dimensional space along a spectrum of possibilities from highly clumped, to independent of each other, to hyper-dispersed. Here we used a Markov Chain not to fit data, but to specify hypothetical situations, in which to try to predict adaptive predator behavior. We called the two kinds of prey mimics and models, after other authors who invented these names (I would have called them tasty and yechy so I could remember which was which). So we denote a mimic with T and a model with Y and describe their distribution in space with a Markov chain. Denote with p the probability that a predator encounters a Y next after encountering a T, and with q the probability that a predator encounters a T next after encountering a Y. The distribution of Y and T in space can be described with a transition matrix:

	T	Y
T	$1 - p$	p
Y	q	$1 - q$

If $p + q = 1$ then Tasties and Yechies occur independently of each other, if $p + q < 1$ then each tends to be clumped together with others of its own kind, and if $p + q > 1$ then the two kinds deliberately mixed together. Thus, the magnitude of $p + q$ measures the intensity and direction of the inter-mixing of prey in this environment. This little Markov chain is a useful tool for modeling environments in which some other question is being studied. The mathematics involved are beyond the scope of this book, but if you are interested in this subject, you are welcome to read our paper, and those that referenced it in the years that followed.

Condor demography

Mertz (1971) published a theoretical analysis of the demography of the endangered California Condor population. California Condors usually give two years of parental care to one young before it leaves the nest to be a self-sufficient juvenile for three more years before becoming a reproductive adult. The probability that baby Condor survives the first year of life is denoted f. If baby Condor does not survive, then its parents will initiate another baby the following year, but if baby Condor does survive then its parents will care for it during the following year and not initiate a another baby until the year after. Breeding adult Condors themselves survive any given year with probability denoted p. Mertz (1971) described this re-nesting behavior as problematic when trying to estimate the number of babies a Condor might initiate in its lifetime, and the number of them that might survive into the second year of parental care. The problem was not solved and mistakes propagated through the literature for a decade and a half (Hoogendyk and Estabrook 1984).

A Markov process can describe this dependency. With it, you can estimate the number of babies a Condor would be expected to initiate in its lifetime, and the number that would be expected to survive into their second year. Once these problematic dependencies have been adequately described by a Markov process, you can use statistical arguments to estimate and compare the demographic parameters. Try to describe this Markov process yourself, then look below to see how I did it.

The Markov process could work like this. In any given year, a parent Condor is dead (D), caring for a child in its first year (F), or be caring for a child in its second year (S). These are the states of the Markov process. The transition matrix is shown below:

	D	F	S
D	1	0	0
F	$1 - p$	$p \times (1 - f)$	$p \times f$
S	$1 - p$	p	0

You can now use this transition matrix to answer the three questions in terms of p and f. This will tell you about Condor survivorship.

9.3   Analysis of covariance

Example

XYZideae, recovered from 19 strata spanning the past 2 million years in roughly 100 000 year increments, have shown very reliable preservation of their gizmos and whizmos. Both gizmo length and whizmo diameter seem to have gotten smaller over time (see opposite):

These are the descriptive regression results for the table below:

GL = 14.408 + 0.781 × time + error
   SSE0 = 370.048   SSE = 22.062
WD = 8.758 + 0.294 × time + error
   SSE0 = 73.512   SSE = 24.223

×100 000 bp	Gizmo length	Whizmo diameter
1	17.000	9.000
2	18.237	9.801
3	16.992	9.981
4	16.843	10.868
5	18.039	10.977
6	18.616	10.643
7	19.144	11.696
8	19.343	11.589
9	20.237	10.690
10	21.179	9.830
11	21.896	9.217
12	22.144	10.996
13	24.835	12.173
14	25.963	11.343
15	25.943	14.433
16	28.191	14.239
17	28.880	15.465
18	28.822	14.474
19	29.905	14.863

Gizmo length is decreasing on average 0.781 per 100 000 yr, and whizmo diameter is decreasing on average 0.294 per 100 000 yr. We already know how to ask whether these rates are different from zero; in this section we will consider how to ask are they different from each other. A natural statistic for this purpose is the rate difference, in this case $|0.781 - 0.294| = 0.487$.

Are the rates equal?

Classical statistics addresses this problem by hypothesizing normal distributions, and comparing estimates of covariance to calculate a complicated statistic with known distribution. For this reason this approach is called analysis of covariance. But to answer the question, Are the rates equal?, we will take a computational approach.

Suppose $GL[t] = GL[t-1] + \mathbf{inc}$, in which **inc** is a random variable that represents the amount by which the size changed (the increment) between time $t-1$ ago and time t ago. If $E(\mathbf{inc})$ is positive then we could say that GL is getting smaller. If $V(\mathbf{inc})$ is low, then GL is getting smaller more consistently. If $V(\mathbf{inc})$ is high, we may not even be able to estimate $E(\mathbf{inc})$ accurately enough to tell whether or not GL's size is getting smaller. We use the observed data to isolate samples of **inc** by subtracting $GL(t-1)$ from $GL(t)$.

A null hypothesis

What could it mean for gizmo length and whizmo diameter NOT to be changing at different rates? They could each be sampling the same increment random variable. We have $18 + 18 = 36$ samples of the random variable, **inc**. They are listed below:

×100 000 bp	GL increment	WD increment
1	1.237	0.801
2	−1.245	0.180
3	−0.149	0.886
4	1.196	0.110
5	0.577	−0.335
6	0.528	1.053
7	0.199	−0.107
8	0.894	−0.899
9	0.942	−0.859
10	0.717	−0.613
11	0.248	1.778
12	2.691	1.177
13	1.128	−0.830
14	−0.020	3.090
15	2.248	−0.194
16	0.689	1.226
17	−0.058	−0.991
18	1.083	0.389

One way to make specific the hypothesis that gizmo length and whizmo diameter are changing at the same rate is to hypothesize that they are both sampling the same **inc** random variable whose distribution is defined by re-sampling the pool of combined observed increments. To simulate data sets under this hypothesis, you re-sample this pool.

Some of the statements in a macro to do this are shown below. The calculation of the value of the observed value of the test statistic, RATEDIF, and place naming and typing are not shown. B1 is named as an array of length 2 so that a single "For K .. Next" loop can re-sample data to simulate both Gismos and Whizmos:

```
For I = 1 To LEN-1
    INCPOOL(2*I-1) = GLINC(I)
    INCPOOL(2*I) = WDINC(I)
    Next I
Randomize
SIGHI = 0
SIGLO = 0
NIP = 2*LEN - 2
Y(1) = 1
For NS = 1 To 1000
  For K = 1 To 2
     For I = 2 To LEN
        X = Rnd * NIP
        J = 1
        Do Until J > X
           J = J + 1
           Loop
        Y(I) = Y(I-1) + INCPOOL(J)
        Next I
     Call LINMO(LEN,X(),Y(),B0,B1(K),SSE,SSE0)
'B1(1) is a simulated Gismo rate, B1(2) a simulated Whizmo rate
     Next K

   SRATEDIF = B1(1) - B1(2) 'Simulated Rate Difference
   If SRATEDIF < 0 Then SRATEDIF = - SRATEDIF
   If SRATEDIF <= RATEDIF Then SIGLO = SIGLO + 1;
   If SRATEDIF >= RATEDIF Then SIGHI = SIGHI + 1;
   Next NS 'End simulations
```

Simulated reality

When this macro was run with the observed data, the realized significances for RATEDIF were SIGHI = 187 and SIGLO = 813, making a very weak suggestion that the rates might be different. In fact, I simulated the data of this example with a macro, like this:

```
Y(1) = 17    'gizmo length
Z(1) = 9     'whizmo diameter
X(1) = 1     'number of 100 000 years before present
LEN = 19
Randomize
For I = 2 To LEN
    X(I) = I
    Call NORMAL(RV)
    'NORMAL samples the (0,1) normal distribution, as in 6.2
    Y(I) = Y(I-1) + 0.3 + RV
    Call NORMAL(RV)
    Z(I) = Z(I-1) + 0.3 + RV
    Next I
```

You can see that the increment is normally distributed with an expected value of 0.3 and a variance of 1.0, and that the observed data themselves were simulated under the hypothesis that the rates are equal. It is important to remember that in statistical arguments equal does not mean exactly equal, it means determined by the same random process. Since the observed-data-simulating macro was already written, I ran it again. What happened is shown next page.

Here are the results when these observations were analyzed:

GL = 14.769 + 0.301 × time + error
SSE0 = 68.084 SSE = 16.506
WD = 8.002 + 0.336 × time + error
SSE0 = 89.822 SSE = 25.587

In this case, when the data were simulated 1000 times, the realized significance of the Whizmo rate minus the Gizmo rate was SIGHI = 932 and SIGLO = 68. This time the rates look statistically almost too similar, as if

×100 000 bp	Gizmo length	Whizmo diameter
1	17.000	9.000
2	16.379	8.494
3	15.086	9.637
4	15.729	10.032
5	16.755	10.228
6	16.040	10.312
7	15.876	9.143
8	16.389	11.369
9	15.517	11.347
10	17.203	11.516
11	18.121	10.758
12	17.676	10.404
13	18.871	10.359
14	19.882	11.926
15	19.155	10.776
16	20.668	14.373
17	21.393	14.698
18	19.980	14.563
19	20.038	16.890

there were some cause keeping them more nearly equal than would be expected if their rate changes were sampling the same random variable. This shows that a statistical argument, whether or not it is made computationally, argues plausibility, but rarely provides proof. If we kept generating observed data sets, we would get one that would reject the hypothesis that the rates are equal, even though in a probabilistic sense they are always equal.

Kitchell *et al.* (1987) provide a published example of this computational approach to analysis of covariance applied to natural data.

9.4   Confounding dependencies

The problem

Sometimes you want to compare a group of big things with a group of little things with respect to something other than size, but you do not want size differences to interfere with your comparison. An example of this situation is sexual dimorphism, in which the males and females of a given species have different average sizes. Suppose you caught and weighed 11 adult squirrels of one species, and 11 adult squirrels of another species. Each species was represented by five females and six males. Their weights, in arbitrary units, are given below:

	Species 1		Species 2	
	Female	Male	Female	Male
	3	6	8	10
	6	4	12	12
	4	5	6	8
	4	5	8	8
	3	4	6	10
		6		12
Average	4	5	8	10
Dimorphism	5/4 = 1.25		10/8 = 1.25	

In this example, Species 2 is twice as big as Species 1, but their sexual dimorphisms (ratio of male to female weight) are the same.

In a real situation, because of natural random variation, even if the sexual dimorphism for two species were the same, you would probably not get exactly the same estimates by weighing samples of males and females from each species. To statistically test the hypothesis that two species have the same sexual dimorphism, you must state the hypothesis in probability terms. I hypothesized that the weights of the females in either species are all independently sampling the same probability distribution, and the weights of the males in either species are all independently sampling the same probability distribution, but not necessarily the same one that the females are sampling. Sexual dimorphism would be the same for each species in the sense that their weights sample the same random variables, but because of this random variation estimates made by weighing squirrels would probably not be exactly the same. How different must the estimates be to credibly argue that the sexual dimorphisms are not the same, i.e., the hypothesis is wrong? The hypothesis predicts a probability distribution for a test statistic to help you answer this question. However, a look at the data above makes it clear that this hypothesis is almost certainly wrong even in a case where sexual dimorphisms are exactly the same. This is because the size difference between the two species is confounding the comparison.

Size-independent units

One way to solve this problem is to change the units of one or both species so that with the new units both species are the same size. This can be done by dividing the weights by their within-species average to express them in units of within-species average. After this has been done, both species have an average weight of 1.0. The average weight of Species 1 is 50/11, and the average weight of Species 2 is 100/11. Dividing each weight by its species-average results in the transformed data below:

	Species 1		Species 2	
	Female	Male	Female	Male
	0.66	1.32	0.88	1.10
	1.32	0.88	1.32	1.32
	0.88	1.10	0.66	0.88
	0.88	1.10	0.88	0.88
	0.66	0.88	0.66	1.10
		1.32		1.32
Average	0.88	1.10	0.88	0.10
Dimorphism	1.10/0.88 = 1.25		1.10/0.88 = 1.25	

You can see that the transformation that expresses the data in units of average species weight does not change the sexual dimorphism, but it does result in two species with the same average weight. The transformed female weights and the male weights may not be sampling the same distributions, as hypothesized to express the idea that the sexual dimorphisms are not different, but if they are not, the reason is no longer because the species are of different average size.

Design a macro

With a natural example, in which the estimated sexual dimorphisms will be different, a relevant test statistic would be the sexual dimorphism of Species 1 minus the sexual dimorphism of Species 2. I wrote a macro to simulate a data set, under the hypothesis that sexual dimorphism is not different in the two species. I pooled the female weights and re-sampled them to create simulated female weights for the two species, and I pooled the male weights and re-sampled them to create simulated male weights for the two species. Then, using these simulated data, I calculated a simulated value for the test statistic. I put all of this in a "For.. Next" loop to repeat it 1000 times to estimate a realized significance for the test statistic.

In this macro, I named and typed at the Module level some of the places I intended to use. This is done at the very beginning, before any procedure, "Sub ()" is defined. Places named at the Module level can be read by any of the statements in the procedures to follow. When different procedures need to read, but not change, the data in a large number of places, it is convenient to name them at the Module level. Names of places whose contents may be changed by a procedure are still best passed in the argument sequence at the time the procedure is called. At the beginning of each "Sub()" in the Module, I used a comment to list as EXTERNAL the Module level places that the statements in this "Sub()" will read. Places I named and typed at the Module level included the weights of males and females of each species, and the numbers of each, together with their averages and observed sexual dimorphisms. I found it convenient for my macro to use two procedures:

```
Sub RANDOM(R As Integer, N As Integer)
    'Loads R equiprobably with an integer between 1 and N
Sub CALCSTAT(TEST As Single) 'Calculate test statistic
```

I named the main "Sub()" that calls these procedures Sub SEXDIMO(). It is the only one I allow to write contents into the places named at the Module level. Especially as programs become more complicated, if you let other procedures change the contents of Module level places it can become extremely difficult to find mistakes.

SEXDIMO reads from "Sheet1" the numbers of males and females of each species, as well as these numbers of weights for each. Note that it is important to read how many weights you need to read before you try to read them. Now the macro is ready to "Call CALCSTAT(STAT)", which calculates average weights and sexual dimorphisms. These are written back to the "Sheet1". Next, the weights are re-scaled to units of species average weight, so that each species has the same average weight. The weight of each individual in these new units is written to "Sheet1". Now the macro makes a list of the weights of females from both species to serve as a female pool to re-sample. It does the same for males. The macro is now ready to simulate 1000 data sets by re-sampling the female pool and the male pool, each time calculating the difference between the sexual dimorphism of species 1 and the sexual dimorphism of species 2, comparing this difference to the observed difference, and incrementing significance counters. Finally significances are written to "Sheet1". These techniques should be familiar to you by now, but if you want to see them again in detail, my complete EXCEL macro to estimate realized significances of the difference in sexual dimorphism is shown in Section 9.5.

Exponential size difference

Often when one species of animal is littler and another is bigger, the bigger species is proportionally bigger. This means that a larger animal of the bigger species tends to differ more in size from a larger animal in the littler species, than does a smaller animal in the bigger species differ from a smaller animal in the littler species. Five females from one species of monkey are heavier than five females from another species, but also a pair of bigger monkeys, one from each species, is more different than a pair of smaller monkeys, one from each species.

	F1	F2
	3.00	4.48
	3.33	5.29
	3.67	6.26
	4.00	7.39
	4.33	8.73
E	3.67	6.43
V	0.22	2.26

Not only are the average sizes different but the larger species is more variable. Dividing each species by its own average, 3.67 and 6.43 respectively, gives the transformed sizes below:

F1	F2
0.82	0.70
0.91	0.82
1.00	0.97
1.09	1.15
1.18	1.36

The average for each species is now 1.00, but their variances are still different, although less so: $V(F1) = 0.017$, $V(F2) = 0.055$. Thus even in units of species average, it does not look like both species could be sampling the same probability distribution.

Differences proportional to size implies exponential growth. This kind of difference can be reversed by logarithmic shrinking, i.e., by transforming the sizes with LN(size). Divide by the average of the transformed sizes of species 2 (1.83) and multiply by the average of original sizes of species 1 (3.67) as shown below:

F1	F2	LN(F2)	LN(F2)×3.67/1.83
3.00	4.48	1.50	3.00
3.33	5.29	1.67	3.33
3.67	6.26	1.83	3.67
4.00	7.39	2.00	4.00
4.33	8.73	2.17	4.33

To make this example, I created the F2 weights as a deterministic exponential function of the F1 weights. With natural data, such a transformation of the larger species will not create an exact copy of the sizes of the smaller species, but if difference is proportional to size, it will create transformed sizes that are comparable enough to pool and re-sample to test hypotheses of dimorphism.

Size difference is part of your hypothesis

It may not be possible to tell with certainty how size differs between two species. One may be proportionally larger than the other, as in the first example above. Size may increase exponentially within species, as in the second example. Although these are two common ways in which size can differ, there are other possibilities, which I will not discuss. To reduce or eliminate the effect of size on comparisons such as sexual dimorphism, you must include in your hypothesis how you suppose that size differs, so you can undo size differences in that way. Many scientists just look at the data and choose a way that size seems to differ, which probably works OK in many cases. You could take a slightly more rigorous approach by ranking the sizes of females (or males) within each species from smallest to largest, then calculate the ratio of larger to smaller species for pairs of monkeys with the same rank for about the first 1/3 of the ranks. Then rank the monkeys from largest to smallest and calculate the ratio of monkeys with the same rank for about the first 1/3 of the ranks. Arrange these in order of size of monkeys with small ranks followed by large ranks. Then fit a regression $Y(i) = B0 + B(1) \times X(i) + E(i)$ where i is a pair of monkeys, $X(i)$ is order, and $Y(i)$ is ratio. If B0 and B1 are not different from 0, then size differs proportionally, as in the first example. If B1 is positive (and B0 is whatever it is), then the larger monkeys of both species differ by a larger factor than do smaller monkeys. In this case, a LN transformation may be more appropriate, as in the second example.

9.5   Sub SEXDIMO

```
'Module level declarations
Dim F1(50) As Single
Dim F2(50) As Single
Dim M1(50) As Single
Dim M2(50) As Single 'Weights of animals
Dim NF1, NF2, NM1, NM2 As Integer 'lengths of the above arrays
Dim AF1, AF2, AM1, AM2 As Single 'AF1 = average weight females
                              'in Species 1, etc
Dim SDM1, SDM2 As Single 'sexual dimorphisms
                          '= ratio of AM1/AF1 or AM2/AF2
Sub RANDOM(R As Integer, N As Integer)
    Dim X As Single      'Load R equiprobably with an integer
    X = Rnd              'between 1 and N
    X = X * N
    R = 1
    Do Until R > X
       R = R + 1
       Loop
End Sub
```

```
Sub CALCSTAT(TEST As Single)
'EXTERNAL NF1,NF2,NM1,NM2,F1(),F2(),M1(),M2(),
'AM1,AM2,AF1,AF2,SDM1,SDM2
    Dim I As Integer
        AM1 = 0#                        'Load TEST with the test statistic
        For I = 1 To NM1
            AM1 = AM1 + M1(I)
            Next I
        AM1 = AM1 / NM1
        AF1 = 0#
        For I = 1 To NF1
            AF1 = AF1 + F1(I)
            Next I
        AF1 = AF1 / NF1
        SDM1 = AM1 / AF1
        AM2 = 0#
        For I = 1 To NM2
            AM2 = AM2 + M2(I)
            Next I
        AM2 = AM2 / NM2
        AF2 = 0#
        For I = 1 To NF2
            AF2 = AF2 + F2(I)
            Next I
        AF2 = AF2 / NF2
        SDM2 = AM2 / AF2

        If SDM1 > SDM2 Then
            TEST = SDM1 - SDM2
        Else
            TEST = SDM2 - SDM1
        End If
    End Sub 'CALCSTAT

Sub SEXDIMO()
Dim I, K As Integer 're-usable indices
Dim J As Integer
Dim MP(100), FP(100) As Single
```

```
                    'pools of combined males, females
Dim TF As Integer 'total number of females in both species
Dim TM As Integer 'total number of males in both species
Dim AW1, AW2 As Single 'average weight of species 1, .. 2
Dim STAT As Single
Dim SSTAT As Single 'test statistic |sdm1-sdm2|
Dim SIGHI, SIGLO, NS As Integer 'significance counters,
                                'number of simulations
MsgBox ("Start")
NF1 = Worksheets("Sheet1").Cells(1,1)
NM1 = Worksheets("Sheet1").Cells(1,2)
NF2 = Worksheets("Sheet1").Cells(1,3)
NM2 = Worksheets("Sheet1").Cells(1,4)

For J = 1 To NF1
    F1(J) = Worksheets("Sheet1").Cells(J + 1,1)
    Next J
For J = 1 To NM1
    M1(J) = Worksheets("Sheet1").Cells(J + 1,2)
    Next J
For J = 1 To NF2
    F2(J) = Worksheets("Sheet1").Cells(J + 1,3)
    Next J
For J = 1 To NM2
    M2(J) = Worksheets("Sheet1").Cells(J + 1,4)
    Next J

Call CALCSTAT(STAT)
Worksheets("Sheet1").Cells(1,5) = AM1
Worksheets("Sheet1").Cells(2,5) = AF1
Worksheets("Sheet1").Cells(3,5) = SDM1
Worksheets("Sheet1").Cells(1,6) = AM2
Worksheets("Sheet1").Cells(2,6) = AF2
Worksheets("Sheet1").Cells(3,6) = SDM2
TF = NF1 + NF2          'Rescale weights in units
TM = NM1 + NM2          'of average species weight
AW1 = 0#
For I = 1 To NF1
    AW1 = AW1 + F1(I)
    Next I
```

```
For I = 1 To NM1
    AW1 = AW1 + M1(I)
    Next I
AW1 = AW1 / (NF1 + NM1)
For I = 1 To NF1
    F1(I) = F1(I) / AW1
    Next I
For I = 1 To NM1
    M1(I) = M1(I) / AW1
    Next I
AW2 = 0#
For I = 1 To NF2
    AW2 = AW2 + F2(I)
    Next I
For I = 1 To NM2
    AW2 = AW2 + M2(I)
    Next I
AW2 = AW2 / (NF2 + NM2)
For I = 1 To NF2
    F2(I) = F2(I) / AW2
    Next I
For I = 1 To NM2
    M2(I) = M2(I) / AW2
    Next I
'Write weights in units of species average weight
'In these units each species has the same average weight
Worksheets("Sheet1").Cells(1,7) = "F1"
Worksheets("Sheet1").Cells(1,8) = "M1"
Worksheets("Sheet1").Cells(1,9) = "F2"
Worksheets("Sheet1").Cells(1,10) = "M2"
For J = 1 To NF1
    Worksheets("Sheet1").Cells(J + 1, 7) = F1(J)
    Next J
For J = 1 To NM1
    Worksheets("Sheet1").Cells(J + 1, 8) = M1(J)
    Next J
For J = 1 To NF2
    Worksheets("Sheet1").Cells(J + 1, 9) = F2(J)
    Next J
```

```
For J = 1 To NM2
    Worksheets("Sheet1").Cells(J + 1,10) = M2(J)
    Next J
For I = 1 To NF1 'Make female and male pools
    FP(I) = F1(I)
    Next I
For I = NF1 + 1 To NF1 + NF2
    FP(I) = F2(I - NF1)
    Next I
For I = 1 To NM1
    MP(I) = M1(I)
    Next I
For I = NM1 + 1 To NM1 + NM2
    MP(I) = M2(I - NM1)
    Next I

MsgBox ("Begin Simulations")
SIGHI = 0
SIGLO = 0
Randomize
For NS = 1 To 1000              'simulate 1000 data sets
For I = 1 To NF1
    Call RANDOM(J, TF)
    F1(I) = FP(J)
    Next I
For I = 1 To NF2
    Call RANDOM(J, TF)
    F2(I) = FP(J)
    Next I

For I = 1 To NM1
    Call RANDOM(J, TM)
    M1(I) = MP(J)
    Next I
For I = 1 To NM2
    Call RANDOM(J, TM)
    M2(I) = MP(J)
    Next I
```

```
        Call CALCSTAT(SSTAT)
        If STAT <= SSTAT Then SIGHI = SIGHI + 1
        If STAT >= SSTAT Then SIGLO = SIGLO + 1
        Next NS
Worksheets("Sheet1").Cells(4,5) = SIGHI
Worksheets("Sheet1").Cells(4,6) = SIGLO
MsgBox ("Done")
End Sub
```

10 | How to get away with peeking at data

Examples

Paulo watched two male *Mus domesticus* (house mouse) interacting to establish dominance. For each 3 second interval, he recorded + if a mouse did a particular behavior, such as groom himself, or − if that behavior was not performed. This sequence was recorded for one of the behaviors of the finally dominant mouse.

$$- - - + - - + - + - - - - + - + - - + - + + - - + - - + + - + - -$$

Paulo wondered if the frequency with which the mouse performed this behavior changed at some point in the interaction; perhaps at the time he began to assume dominance. So Paulo looked through the data sequence for the time when the difference between the frequency before and the frequency after is the greatest. Then he used the hypothesis that the behavior is performed independently with the same probability for each interval to test if the frequency with which the behavior is performed before this time is different from that after this time. Somehow, he was not surprised that these frequencies turned out to be significantly different. After all, he peeked at the sequence to divide it at the point of maximal difference.

Jennifer and her colleagues observed fossil Forams (little shelled animals that lived at the bottom of the sea hundreds of millions of years ago) that had changed size through evolutionary time. Looking at a plot of size vs time before present, Forams seemed to be getting bigger. In addition, the plot of points seemed to bend at a particular time in the past, suggesting that the rate of increase after that time was more rapid. Had the evolutionary rate changed at that time? So they used the computational ANCOVA technique, described in Section 9.3, to test for equality of rate before and after that time. Somehow, they were not surprised that the rates were different. After all, they had peeked at the data to find the time before and after which rate difference was greatest.

Recall David's *Amelanchier arboria* data, from Section 2.3. He wanted to test the idea that a single probability for seed mortality could account for the observed pattern, if the empty carpels that corresponded to carpel paired mortality of both seeds were removed. But he did not know which of the 55 empty carpels these were. So he removed empty carpels until the goodness of fit to the binomial distribution of number of carpels with 2, 1, or 0 seeds was maximized. Recall that David observed 215 carpels, of which 91 had 2 seeds, 69 had 1, and 55 had 0. The subsequent statistical test of goodness of fit to the binomial distribution failed to reject the binomial distribution. But he was not very convinced by this, because, after all, he had altered the data to give the best fit.

I weighed the seeds from a flowering head of *Tragopogon dubious* (looks like a big dandelion). These are my seed weights in grams:

6.0   5.6   5.4   5.1   4.7   4.4   4.1   3.6   3.3   3.1   2.8   2.5   2.2   1.8

I wondered if *Tragopogon dubius* were making two sizes of seeds (with variation), lighter seeds near the top of the seed head that blow away under their parachutes (like dandelion), and heavier seeds lower down that catch with little hooks on the fur of animals. The lighter seeds would be more likely to blow far away, and the heavier seeds more likely to disperse locally. To test this idea, I divided the seeds into two groups: the seven heaviest seeds and the seven lightest seeds. Then I tested to see if these two groups differ in weight, using a program to test the difference between two groups, similar to the one that you wrote in Section 2.5, to help Patricia compare bird weights. I was not surprised that the two groups turned out to be significantly different; after all I sorted them into the big seed group and the small seed group before I tested for their difference.

The problem

In every case, the statistical technique, even though computational, seemed unconvincing because the investigators had peeked at the data to hypothesize something related to what they had seen. Whether or not the hypothesized processes were operative, peeking at the data makes it more likely that a statistical test will support the argument the investigator wants to make, because the data were structured, or a hypothesis was chosen, to favor a particular answer to the question being asked. The examples above are flagrant, but there are subtler ways for peeking at the data to influence the design of statistical tests, so it is important to watch for them. Normally, peeking weakens or invalidates your statistical argument.

Classical statistics can recognize some instances of peeking and deal with them effectively. For example, when you use the average of several samples of a normally distributed random variable to estimate its mean, and then use that estimate of mean to estimate its variance, you peeked at the sampled data and used the knowledge gained (your estimate of mean) to estimate variance. Variance is the expected squared deviation from the distribution mean. Recall that for a collection of samples, the sum of squared deviations from some number is minimized when that number is the sample average. But the distribution mean is almost always different from the sample average. Thus, using the sum of the sample squared deviations from the sample average to estimate variance almost always underestimates variance. The mathematics of classical statistics have shown that in the case of normal distributions, you can correct for the underestimate. i.e., make an unbiased estimator, by dividing by $(n - 1)$ instead of by n, the sum of squared deviations from the sample average. Also, you can get away with peeking at the mean in comparisons of variance estimates by reducing the apparent degrees of freedom, m, by 1, to get $(m - 1)$, in Chi Square (and consequent) F distributions.

Legitimate peeking

Incorporating suggestions made by the observed data could be legitimate and useful in more general cases, which a computational approach can accommodate. The key to making peeking legitimate is to put the peeking process right into the mechanism that is hypothesized to explain the observed data. In this way the peeking itself is simulated along with the rest of the explanation to calculate the predicted distribution for the test statistic.

Include peeking in your hypothesis

To analyze the data he had gathered watching mice interact, Paulo hypothesized that the probability with which a behavior occurs is the same for each time interval, and is independent of what occurs in other time intervals. He estimated this hypothesized constant probability using an estimating random variable whose value is the number of observed +s divided by number of time intervals, in this example 12/33. This in itself might look like peeking. However, his question is not about the frequency with which a behavior occurs over the whole sequence, but about a possible change in frequency. Using his data to choose this probability ensures that simulated data sets resemble the observed one in a way not directly related to the question of interest. In Section 3.2, 21 ups and 21 downs in the sequence of extinction rates of marine families were observed. Thus, simulating data with 21 ups and 21 downs is more convincing. I wrote a program for my colleague Paulo, which used "If (Rnd * 33 <= 12)" to simulate the occurrence of a behavior. The program did this 33 times to simulate a behavior sequence. Then it peeked at each interval in the middle half of the simulated sequence to discover the one before which, and after which, the simulated frequencies differ the most. This maximum difference is the test statistic. The predicted probability distribution of this peeking statistic is estimated by simulating 1000 behavioral sequences. In this way the peeking to choose the apparent time for frequency switch was hypothesized as well, which makes the predicted distribution a credible basis for argument, even after peeking.

My colleague Jennifer wanted to test her idea about change of evolutionary rates in Forams. So I wrote a program for her that simulates a hypothesis that incorporates peeking. It re-sampled rate increments to create simulated data showing evolutionary change through time. To peek at the simulated data to find the time when evolutionary rates differed the most, for each time interval throughout the middle half of the period studied, my program divided the whole period into two sub-periods, ending or beginning after that time interval. Then my program fit a linear model to each sub-interval and recorded the difference in their B1s. Recall that B1 indicates the rate of evolutionary change. The maximum of these differences is the simulated value of the test statistic. The predicted probability distribution for this greatest difference is estimated by repeating this whole process 1000 times. Now the observation of the apparent time of rate change is part of the random mechanism defined by the hypothesis. It participates in the simulation process so that the predicted distribution for the test statistic includes peeking. Now, this test statistic and its predicted distribution becomes a credible basis for argument.

To test my seed weight idea, I need a hypothesis that incorporates sorting seed weights into heaviest and lightest. The heaviest seven seeds have a mean weight of 5.04, the lightest seven have a mean weight of 2.76 and all 14 have a mean weight of 3.90. The difference between the heavy mean and the light mean is 2.28. How surprised would I be to observe a mean difference of 2.28 if these 14 seed weights were sampling the same distribution? But what same distribution? Because my macro will sort simulated seed weights into heaviest seven and lightest seven to calculate a simulated value for the test statistic, a hypothesis based on permutation would never produce a result different from the observed. Re-sampling would produce results with a little variation, but re-sampling with only 14 observations will not produce much variation for this kind of test statistic either. If the plant developed seed weight by a process analogous to sampling a seed weight random variable many times independently, then the seed weight distribution would approximate a normal distribution. So I chose the normal distribution with mean 3.90 (seed weight sample average), and variance 1.81 (unbiased estimate using sample average) to be the distribution hypothesized to have been sampled by all seed weights. I wrote a macro to: (1) use this hypothesis to simulate 14 seed weights, and (2) then divide them into the heaviest seven and lightest seven and calculate the difference in the means. My macro predicted the distribution for this test statistic by sampling it in this way 1000 times. Now the peeking in the guise of pre-sorting into the heaviest seven and lightest seven has been simulated as well, so that the distribution predicted for the test statistic incorporates peeking and thus becomes a credible basis for argument.

The idea that *Tragopogon dubius* might have evolved to adaptively produce two different seed sizes is interesting; if the data permit, I would like to be able to argue a stronger case. Perhaps *T. dubius* produces any of its possible seed sizes with equal probability. If this hypothesis could be rejected, it would strengthen the argument that *T. dubius* has a proximal mechanism to produce smaller and larger seeds. This hypothesis predicts fewer medium-sized seeds than does the hypothesis based on the normal distribution, so I would need a clearer pattern of big and small seeds to reject it convincingly. I hypothesized that the seed weights sampled a uniform distribution. Because the observed range is (1.8 – 6.0), I hypothesized that seed weights sampled **u**[1.8,6.0]. I wrote a macro to sample this distribution to simulate 14 seed weights, then divide them into the heaviest seven and lightest seven and calculate the difference in the means. This is the same test statistic that I used with the hypothesis based on the normal distribution, but now it has a different predicted distribution. If this peeking-based test statistic rejects the hypothesis based on the normal distribution, I can make a case for two seed sizes. If it also rejects the hypothesis based on this uniform distribution, I can make an even stronger case.

Goodness-of-fit

If you wanted to avoid a peeking-based test statistic, in this case you could take a goodness-of-fit approach to testing this idea, as described in Section 8.2. With only 14 samples, two thresholds making three groups is about as fine as I wanted, so as not to lose power. For the normal distribution hypothesized above, with mean 3.90 and variance 1.81, five observed seed weights fall between plus (4.24) and minus (2.56), one standard deviation (1.34) from the mean. Recall from Section 6.2 that the statements:

$$X = Rnd$$
$$X = 0.603 \times Log(X/(1 - X))$$

sample a normally distributed random variable with mean 0.0 and variance 1.0. To sample the normal-distribution seed-weight hypothesis above, I needed to first multiply X by the standard deviation of the distribution I want to sample (1.34) and then add the mean (3.90), like this

$$X = X \times 1.34$$
$$X = X + 3.9$$

Now X is a simulated seed weight. My program did this 14 times, testing each time whether this simulated weight fell in the interval (4.24, 2.56), and if so incremented a counter. This counter was compared to 5 (the observed number of seeds in this interval), and SIGHI and SIGLO were incremented appropriately. My program did this 1000 times to estimate the realized significance of five seeds in this middle interval. If there are improbably few observed seeds in this middle interval, then I can argue that T. dubius makes big and little seeds.

Some of my students complain that although this text explains how to solve the problems, it usually does not give the answers, i.e., the realized significances of the test statistics in the context of the example data. By now, if you have practiced with the concepts and the programming techniques, copied the examples, and done the exercises, you can write your own macros to get answers. If you want to know these answers, write and run your own macros to find them. But more importantly, now you can ensure that your own statistical arguments are convincing to yourself, and to your colleagues who understand this approach to scientific argument.

11 | Contingency

11.1 What is contingency?

Examples

Birds of a feather nest together, or do they? A pond has three islands where three different species of birds nest. Bird watchers observed the 5 nests on one island, the 8 nests on another island, and the 12 nests on a third island. Of these 25 nests, 10 belonged to birds of species A, 8 to birds of species B, and 7 to birds of species C. Do birds of the same species tend to nest on the same island?

I study culturally informed technology in the context of traditional Portuguese agriculture. As recently as the middle of the twentieth century, in many of the agricultural villages in the mountainous interior of the Beira Alta region of Portugal, virtually all the land was still owned by a few wealthy families. They rented large parcels to farming families, on a more or less permanent basis. These renters owned their own traction animals and equipment and managed their farm, but hired members of the many remaining families to work for them, on a daily basis, to perform much of the farm labor. These day-workers could work for any farmer who would hire them, usually in their own village, but sometimes also in other villages. I wondered if day-workers in the same family tended to work for the same farmer, or for any farmer, or avoided working for the same farmer as other family members.

While conducting research for her Ph.D. thesis, Virginia examined the few known skeletal remains of Neanderthals, humans who lived 130 thousand to 30 thousand years ago in Europe and the Near East, for evidence of healed broken bones. Healed broken bones can be seen in different places in the body: head, arms, trunk, legs, etc. She compared Neanderthals to more modern hunter/gatherer societies by looking for evidence of healed broken bones in their skeletal remains. She wanted to know if Neanderthals tended to break bones in the same parts of their bodies as did these other societies.

Carl found documents from seventeenth century Bristol, England that recorded instances of craftsmen fathers arranging apprenticeships for their young sons, with other master craftsmen. The documents indicated the craft of the father and the craft of the master to whom the son was apprenticed. Carl wanted to know if fathers practicing a given craft tended to apprentice their sons to learn some particular same or other craft.

Substantively, these are very different questions: they come from studies in ecology, cultural anthropology, biological anthropology, and history. However, they all share the same basic data structure for organizing data to prepare to answer the question asked, and they all have relatively small amounts of available data. So they can all be addressed with the same concepts for arguing the relevance of the relationships in question.

Contingency table

In every case, the observations and associated question can be construed as a contingency: there are some things that have been observed (bird's nests, farm laborers, human bones, documents reporting the apprenticeships of young sons), and for each there are two ways to classify those things (islands and species of birds, families and employers, parts of body and Neanderthal vs more modern hunter-gatherer, craft of father and craft of apprentice master). The observed data for such contingencies can be arranged in a two-dimensional table whose rows represent the classes of one classification and whose columns represent the classes of the other classification. Each box of the table is in a particular row and column. It contains the count of the number of cases (nests, laborers, broken bones, apprenticed sons) that are in the class of its row for the row classification, and also in the class of its column for the column classification. When counts have been arrayed in a table like this, called a contingency table, the number of cases in the boxes in each row can be counted to determine the number of things in each class of the row classification. Similarly, the number of cases in each class of the column classification can be determined by counting the number of cases in the boxes in each column.

Independence

The basic question, Are the two classifications independent of each other?, asks whether the probability that something belongs to a given class of one classification changes if it is known to belong to a given class of the other classification? One way to answer this question is to hypothesize that the answer is no. This means that the two classifications are independent. One way to make this hypothesis explicit is to hypothesize that: (1) the probability that a case would be in a class of the row classification is proportional to the frequency with which cases were observed in that class, (2) the probability that a case would be in a class of the column classification is proportional to the frequency with which cases were observed in that class, and (3) once a case was known to belong to a class of one classification, the probabilities with which it belongs to any class of the other classification do not change. Under this hypothesis, the expected value of the count in each box is the number of things in its row class times the number of things in its column class divided by the total number of things.

Goodness-of-fit

In Section 8.2, I talked about testing goodness of fit with a statistic whose distribution would asymptotically approach a parametric Chi Square distribution under the hypothesis that the observed data were in fact samples of the distribution whose goodness of fit was being tested. In the opinion of many scientists, the distribution of this statistic would approach a parametric Chi Square distribution closely enough to support a statistical argument, if enough samples had been observed to ensure that the expected number of samples in each interval was at least 5.0. This same classical approach can be used to test this hypothesis of independence of the row and column classifications of a contingency, when there are enough data to ensure that the expected value of each box is at least 5.0. Recall that the second feature shared by the substantively different examples above is that they each have very little data available with which to argue the differential credibility of competing hypotheses, i.e., the expected values of the counts in their contingency tables are mostly very much less than 5.0.

Useful statistics

With a computational approach to statistical argument, this is not an insurmountable problem. You can simulate a hypothesis to accurately estimate the probability distribution(s) and realized significance(s) for one or more appropriate test statistics, and make statistical arguments based on them. Contingency provides a data structure and a hypothesis. What should be the test statistics? The problem with the classical Chi Square statistic, described in Section 8.2, is that for small amounts of data, no parametric Chi Square distribution approximates very well the probability distribution of the Chi Square statistic. But now, with the computational techniques described, you can write a macro to simulate a probability distribution that accurately approximates the distribution for a Chi Square (or any other) statistic calculated from a contingency table. What other statistics might be useful? When the Chi Square statistic indicates that the whole table is not consistent with a hypothesis of independence, it would be useful to know which boxes have counts that are inconsistently too high or too low. With a computational approach, every count in the table could be a statistic.

ACTUS

In the late 1980s, I wrote a program to implement these ideas. My brother Carl, with his apprentice data, helped me design a program we called ACTUS (Analysis of Contingency Tables Using Simulation). In the late 1990s I wrote a new version, ACTUS2, to implement some hypotheses of dependency to use with contingency tables. A brief history of ACTUS, and a more detailed explanation of how to use ACTUS2 is given in the next section. To use with my course, I recently wrote a spreadsheet version of ACTUS using two different hypotheses of independence. I explain how to use the spreadsheet version of ACTUS in Section 11.3. Section 11.4 is Sub ACTUS(), the macro statements that implement the version of Section 11.3, using only the programming language and techniques that I have presented in this book, so by now, you should be able to understand it easily.

11.2   ACTUS2

Analysis of contingency tables using simulation

Many scholars, especially those working in museums or archives with limited material, need to analyze contingencies based on very few cases. The approach of classical statistics based on the Chi Square family of distributions is not very accurate in such cases. In the late 1980s, Carl (my brother and a professor of history at Dartmouth College) and I designed a program to implement a computational approach. We called it ACTUS (Analysis of Contingency Tables Using Simulation) and published its description (Estabrook and Estabrook 1989).

Our original program implemented the hypothesis and the statistics described in the previous section. It was written in PASCAL for a DOS operating system, and was distributed, together with a description of how to use it, to anyone who asked for it. ACTUS came to the attention of some researchers who wanted to use a more restrictive hypothesis of independence, in which the row totals and column totals in simulated tables were always the same as in the observed table. Other researchers, studying animal behavior, encountered contingency tables in which the counts in some of the boxes had to be zero, e.g., for some of the row classes, things in them could not belong to some of the column classes. This results in a hypothesis of partial dependency of the columns on the rows. So, in the late 1990s I wrote a second version, ACTUS2, that implemented both hypotheses of independence and this class of hypotheses of partial dependence.

ACTUS2 was written in PASCAL for DOS operating systems, and also posted on my programs website, http://www-Personal.umich.edu/ ~gfe/ where anyone can download it. I also posted a document giving a much more detailed explanation of how to use ACTUS2, both conceptually and technically. Below is the conceptual part of that document. I omitted the technical parts explaining how to run ACTUS2 in DOS, because that is no longer relevant. By the mid-1990s, nearly all scholars used personal computers with graphic user interfaces, such as Apple OS or WINDOWS, so Borland's Delphi was used to convert the PASCAL version of ACTUS2 into a WINDOWS application. This WINDOWS version implements only the hypotheses of independence. Some of the features of ACTUS2 are described and illustrated in Estabrook (2002).

Exvotos example

In the fall of 1997 I observed a number of small paintings (exvotos) from rustic chapels in the interior of Portugal, painted by local residents to fulfill promises made to saints. They typically depict people experiencing accidents or enduring sickness, in the presence of other people. The paintings were probably made in the nineteenth century. Of the people in these paintings, 52 were apparently female. They can be sorted into classes according to the color of their upper garment. They can also be sorted into classes according to their maturity. We can show the observed relationship between these two ways to classify the women in these paintings by using a two-way contingency in which the columns represent garment color and the rows represent maturity.

The column labels are:	The row labels are:
Col 1: White (Tan)	Row 1: Babies
Col 2: Yellow	Row 2: Children
Col 3: Green	Row 3: Teenagers
Col 4: Blue	Row 4: Middle Aged Women
Col 5: Red	Row 5: Old Women
Col 6: K Black	

The array below contains in each box the number of these 52 females who wear an upper garment (called hereafter a blouse) the color of the column label, and exhibit the maturity of the row label, of the column and row in which that box occurs. As a reminder the first letter of its label is associated with each row or column.

	W	Y	G	B	R	K
B	0	0	0	1	1	0
C	2	3	0	0	1	3
T	9	1	6	3	0	1
M	1	0	1	2	0	1
O	6	1	2	0	0	7

I would like to be able to use these counts, which represent the co-occurrences of maturity and blouse color, to discover whether and how maturity and blouse color are related to each other in this context. One possibility is that they are not related at all.

Under such a hypothesis the column (the blouse color) in which a case (an image of a female person in one of these paintings) occurs does not influence (is independent of) the row (the maturity) in which that case occurs. If such a hypothesis were in fact true, any explanation of why a particular combination of blouse color and maturity might co-occur as frequently or as infrequently as observed would NOT be warranted by the pattern of observed co-occurrences. In this case, it would be a methodological error to present an explanation.

To determine how consistent are the observed counts with a hypothesis that the rows and columns are independent, ACTUS2 uses such a hypothesis to simulate contingency arrays that are examples of what counts could be if the rows and columns were independent. By simulating a large number (1000 or more) of arrays, I can see which (if any) of the observed counts are surprisingly large or small under that hypothesis of independence.

Results of these simulations are presented in two arrays, each with as many rows and columns as observed. One is called the SMALL array; it identifies boxes in the observed array that have a smaller number of cases than would be predicted by that hypothesis of independence. The other is called the BIG array; it identifies boxes in the observed array that have a bigger number of cases than would be predicted by that hypothesis of independence.

SMALL and BIG arrays

This is how ACTUS2 creates the SMALL and BIG arrays. For each simulated array, the count of cases in a given box is compared to the count of cases in the corresponding box of the observed array. After ACTUS2 has simulated 1000 arrays, the number in a given box of the SMALL array is the number of simulated arrays with a count of cases in the given box less than or equal to the count of cases observed in that box. Below is an example of a SMALL array created by ACTUS2 for the observed counts above, under a hypothesis that blouse color and maturity are independent. In each box is the number of simulated arrays out of 1000 in which the count for that box was less than or equal to the observed count for that box:

SMALL ARRAY

	W	Y	G	B	R	K
B	503	830	702	817	998	919
C	376	989	198	418	957	810
T	851	428	929	866	475	32
M	464	600	780	988	829	668
O	696	547	487	211	550	948

Only 32 of every 1000 arrays simulated under that hypothesis of independence have a count of teenagers wearing black that is ≤ 1 (the one teenager among the 52 females in the paintings observed to be wearing black). This suggests that one teenager observed to be wearing black is fewer than would be predicted by that hypothesis of independence. Such an infrequent co-occurrence may warrant explanations based on cultural or historical context.

Similarly, the number in a given box of the BIG array is the number of simulated arrays with a count of cases in that box greater than or equal to the count of cases observed in that box. Below is an example of a BIG array created by ACTUS2 for the observed counts above, under a hypothesis that blouse color and maturity are independent. In each box is the number of arrays (in every 1000 simulated) in which the count for that box was greater than or equal to the observed count for that box.

BIG ARRAY

	W	Y	G	B	R	K
B	1000	1000	1000	1000	104	375
C	832	50	1000	1000	274	393
T	260	844	155	317	1000	995
M	835	1000	592	69	1000	697
O	462	802	778	1000	1000	95

These simulations suggest that the largest observed count is the three children wearing yellow. Only an average of 50 in each 1000 simulated arrays had counts of three or more children wearing yellow. Only 50 such simulated arrays indicate that the count of three children in yellow is higher than would be predicted by that hypothesis of independence. Such frequent co-occurrences may warrant explanations based on cultural or historical context.

Notice that the largest observed count, the nine teenagers in white, is not larger than predicted by this independence hypothesis because nine or more teenagers wore white in more than a quarter of the simulated arrays. Similarly none of the combinations of maturity and blouse color unrepresented by the 52 females in these paintings, indicated by zeros in boxes in the array of observed counts, is smaller than predicted by this independence hypothesis.

Important questions

- There already is a well-known, standard statistical technique using the Chi Square distribution for analyzing contingencies like this one. Why do we need another method?
- ACTUS2 tells us how many simulated arrays have counts in any box less/ greater than or equal to the observed counts. How few such simulated arrays should we have to warrant substantive explanations for low (or high) co-occurrences?
- I have talked of a hypothesis of independence. Can there be more than one?
- Could ACTUS2 analyze a contingency under a hypothesis that specified some dependencies among rows and columns?
- How do you actually use the ACTUS2 computer program?

Significance of the whole contingency

A standard statistical technique using a Chi Square distribution for analyzing contingency does exist to determine whether the hypothesis that the rows and columns (shirt color and maturity) are independent can be rejected. I described it in Section 8.2, when discussing goodness of fit. The value of a Chi Square statistic can also be calculated for this contingency, but there are often three problems with this approach:

(1) The approximation to a Chi Square distribution is not very accurate unless the number of cases expected under the hypothesis of independence is at least 5 for most of the boxes of the contingency. When cases are few, such as in this example, the expected value for many boxes is well below 5. By simulation, ACTUS2 estimates the significance of counts accurately, even with only a few cases.

(2) When a classical statistical Chi Square test tells you that the number of cases in some boxes CAN be interpreted as more (less) frequent than predicted by independence, it is often difficult to tell which boxes they are. As you have seen, ACTUS2 is explicit.

(3) We may be experts in our own fields, but not know the assumptions the mathematical theory on which Chi Square distributions are based, so

using them can be intellectually uncomfortable. ACTUS2 is intellectually accessible, so that we can use it responsibly and with confidence in our scholarship.

The Chi Square statistic is calculated as part of classical statistical techniques. Its possible values approximate a member of the Chi Square family of distributions when, for each box, the counts expected under a hypothesis of independence are large enough; most scientists accept as adequate expected values of at least 5. With fewer cases, the Chi Square statistic could still be a useful indication of the extent to which the counts in the whole array differed from the counts predicted by a hypothesis, if the real distribution for this statistic were known. So ACTUS2 calculates the value of the Chi Square statistic for every simulated array and compares it to the value calculated from the observed array. The fraction of simulated arrays with values greater than or equal to the observed value estimates the realized significance of the observed value of the Chi Square statistic. ACTUS2 reports this fraction, which also depends on the hypothesis used to simulate.

If the whole array does not differ significantly from what would be predicted under the specified hypothesis, then you are not clearly warranted to interpret any of the boxes indicated by the BIG or SMALL arrays. In the example here, there are 30 boxes; if the counts were generated by independent samples of the rows and columns, then one box with unusually few or unusually many cases would not be unusual. If the whole contingency differs significantly from what the specified hypothesis predicts, then you can interpret individual boxes with more confidence.

Under a hypothesis of independence, the counts expected in the boxes of the observed contingency are calculated as the product of the number of cases in the row of the box times the number of cases in the column of the box divided by the total number of cases. Typically, expected counts are fractional, and so are not possible as observed values, which have to be whole numbers. In this sense, they are not expected at all, but they may be of interest. ACTUS2 reports expected counts, as shown below for this example, together with row frequencies RF and column frequencies CF.

Report of expected values

	W	Y	G	B	R	K	RF
B	0.7	0.20	0.3	0.2	0.1	0.5	2
C	3.1	0.9	1.6	0.9	0.3	2.3	9
T	6.9	1.9	3.5	1.9	0.8	5.0	20
M	1.7	0.5	0.9	0.5	0.2	1.3	5
O	5.5	1.5	2.8	1.5	0.6	4.0	16
CF	18	5	9	5	2	13	52

ACTUS2 also reports the deviations between the observed counts and their expected values, as shown below for our example. Negative numbers indicate the extent to which observed counts fell below their expected values. For each box, the sum of the expected value plus the deviation equals the observed count.

	W	Y	G	B	R	K
B	−0.7	−0.2	−0.3	−0.2	−0.9	0.5
C	−1.1	2.1	−1.6	−0.9	0.7	0.8
T	2.1	−0.9	2.5	1.1	−0.8	−4.0
M	−0.7	−0.5	0.1	1.5	−0.2	−0.3
O	0.5	−0.5	−0.8	−1.5	−0.6	3.0

The Chi Square statistic is calculated by a formula involving deviations and expected values. The formula is somewhat complicated because it has been constructed to approximate a member of the Chi Square family of distributions when expected values are high enough, i.e., many cases have been observed in each row and column. ACTUS2 uses the same formula to calculate a value for the Chi Square statistic for every simulated data set. In the example here, these values were equal to or exceeded 40.771 (the value of the Chi Square statistic calculated from the observed counts) 81 times out of 10 000. This shows that the observed value of the Chi Square statistic is high with an estimated realized significance of 0.0081, indicating that the observed counts are not at all consistent with the specified hypothesis of independence. The high or low counts revealed by the SMALL and BIG arrays can be interpreted with some confidence that they would not occur very often at random or by chance.

ACTUS2 compares the value of a statistic calculated from the observed counts with its value calculated in the same way from simulated counts. It estimates the realized significance of the statistic with the fraction of simulated arrays for which its value is not less (or not greater) than its observed value. This works for any statistic, not just those that approximate a known pre-calculated distribution. So, ACTUS2 also uses an easy-to-understand, direct measure of the extent to which an observed contingency differs from the expected values predicted by a specified hypothesis. This statistic is called SAD (the Sum of the Absolute values of the Differences between the expected values and the observed values). SAD is calculated by adding the deviations, without their minus signs. In our example, the values of SAD calculated for each simulated array of counts was equal to or exceeded 31.538 (the value calculated from the observed counts) 87 times out of 10 000.

The realized significance of statistics such as Chi Square or SAD also depends on the hypothesis that predicts their distribution. Usually, when ACTUS2 makes computational estimates of the significances of SAD and of the Chi Square statistic, they are close. They both indicate whether the contingency as a whole warrants interpretation. SAD is more readily understood than the Chi Square statistic, but calculates something slightly different; it gives less weight to boxes with large deviations from expected.

Interpret significance

How few simulated arrays with values greater (less) than or equal to those observed in a given box are required to indicate that an observed count is sufficiently small or big to be interpreted substantively? The counts of simulated arrays of counts shown in the SMALL and BIG arrays are the realized significances of the corresponding observed counts, under the specified hypothesis. ACTUS2 shows them in units of 1000, even though 10 000 arrays are simulated. This makes the results easier to read, and 1000 is more than enough precision to make scientific arguments with these realized significances. Divide the counts reported by 1000 to get a p value. What value of p indicates that a box in the observed contingency can be credibly interpreted as rejecting the specific hypothesis? The answer depends on what you and other scholars in your field consider convincing. Many scientists accept that boxes whose counts have a significance below

5 percent, i.e., SMALL or BIG array entries less than or equal to 50, can be plausibly interpreted. Significances above 10 percent indicate that the observed count is equalled or exceeded among simulated arrays so often that it might be consistent with the specified hypothesis, so that no other explanation is warranted.

Remember that these guidelines refer to a single test. In a contingency, many boxes are potentially interpretable. For this reason it is important to use the significance of the whole contingency as a guide. If the SAD or Chi Square significance is above the 5 percent level, individual boxes should be interpreted more cautiously. When the whole contingency has a significance well above 5 percent, do not interpret individual boxes.

Often a contingency will differ significantly from the predictions of a specified hypothesis if many boxes are consistently somewhat high or somewhat low. With a very significant whole array, several boxes with individual levels of significance between 5 and 10 percent can be interpreted as trends, in the opinion of many scientists.

Estimated significances are especially important as indicators of what NOT to interpret, especially with few cases. As we have seen, the nine teenagers in white is the largest entry in the array of counts, but nine is not surprisingly large under this hypothesis of independence. The seven old ladies in black may warrant interpretation (in this culture widows wear black) but the count of six old ladies in white would be typical if age and dress color were not related. Thus, some of the largest observed counts should not be interpreted as large, and not any of the 11 zeros and only one of the 8 ones might be interpreted as small.

Another hypothesis of independence

The explanations above refer to a hypothesis of independence. A hypothesis is specified in sufficient detail that it can be simulated unambiguously, when it is clear exactly how to generate a data set at random. Such a clarification consists of listing, or describing, the possible choices, and then for each one stating the probability of choosing it. This clarification is an important part of the hypothesis because different procedures for choosing at random can result in different predictions. In the case of ACTUS2, this could result in identifying different boxes for interpretation.

One hypothesis of independence that ACTUS2 can use is called Hypothesis F because it chooses at random based on frequencies. Hypothesis F defines the probability that a simulated case occurs in a given column to be proportional to the frequency of observed cases in that column. The probability that the same simulated case occurs in a given row is defined to be proportional to the frequency of observed cases in that row. By means of a random number generator, ACTUS2 uses these probabilities to independently select a row and column for as many simulated cases as there were observed cases. This generates a simulated array of co-occurrences.

The other hypothesis of independence that ACTUS2 can use is called Hypothesis P because it chooses at random based on permutations. A permutation of the observed cases is a possible ordering of them from first to last. Hypothesis P defines the probability of each possible permutation of the observed cases to be equally likely. To assign columns to simulated cases, one of these permutations is chosen at random. Starting with the first case, as many cases are assigned to column 1 as there are observed cases in column 1. Continuing with the next case, as many cases are assigned to column 2 as there are observed cases in column 2. This process continues for any remaining columns until all cases to be simulated have been assigned a column. In this way, the simulated columns are assigned independently of the observed rows, which remain the same in the simulated array as was observed. Under hypothesis P, the numbers of cases in the rows and columns of a simulated array are always the same as the numbers of observed cases in the corresponding rows and columns, which is not usually the case under hypothesis F.

No matter which hypothesis is chosen, rows and columns are assigned to simulated cases independently, and each simulated array has the same number of cases as were observed. Many more different possible simulated arrays can be created under hypothesis F than under hypothesis P, which allows for many fewer possibilities. Keeping the row and column sums the same as observed may be considered a desirable quality of the P hypothesis. If the totality of things representing cases can be considered all that ever were, then the P hypothesis might be considered the most appropriate. However, the F hypothesis simulates contingencies that may more realistically represent a random collection of a few cases, such as those in an archive or museum, from the many that were extant. Among these simulated arrays might be included, some quite unlike the one actually observed, but similar to tables that represent samples of all the cases. Often results from the two hypotheses are similar, varying in degree (as this example will show).

Below is the SMALL array from our example, made under the F hypothesis, followed by a SMALL array made under the P hypothesis.

A SMALL array under hypothesis F:

	W	Y	G	B	R	K
B	503	830	802	817	998	919
C	376	989	198	418	957	810
T	851	428	929	866	475	32
M	464	600	780	988	829	668
O	696	547	487	211	550	948

A SMALL array under hypothesis P:

	W	Y	G	B	R	K
B	407	817	708	831	997	947
C	329	996	148	393	979	854
T	926	365	986	940	567	5
M	429	579	809	995	799	621
O	754	509	417	138	501	995

Below is the BIG array for this example, made under hypothesis F. It is followed by a BIG array made under hypothesis P.

A BIG array under hypothesis F:

	W	Y	G	B	R	K
B	1000	1000	1000	1000	104	375
C	832	50	1000	1000	274	393
T	260	844	155	317	1000	995
M	835	1000	592	69	1000	697
O	462	802	778	1000	1000	95

A BIG array under hypothesis P:

	W	Y	G	B	R	K
B	1000	1000	1000	1000	74	461
C	891	31	1000	1000	344	386
T	199	916	74	261	1000	999
M	881	1000	623	80	1000	785
O	478	878	846	1000	1000	43

The difference between these results is essentially one of degree. The number of teenagers wearing black was significantly small under hypothesis F, but very significantly small under hypothesis P. Because hypothesis P always keeps the simulated row and column totals the same as observed, many fewer different arrays can be simulated. If it is important to the substantive argument to test for independence of row and column classifications under a hypothesis that keeps the number of cases in the simulated arrays the same as in the observed array, then hypothesis P would be preferred.

The BIG table results are similar, but under hypothesis P, old women in black and children in yellow are more significantly interpretable. Because hypothesis P always keeps the simulated row and column totals the same as observed, many fewer different arrays can be simulated. If it is important to the substantive argument to test for independence of row and column classifications under a hypothesis that keeps the number of cases in the simulated arrays the same as in the observed array, then hypothesis P would be preferred.

The whole contingency has a realized significance under F of about 0.01 for both Chi Square and SAD, and under P of about 0.005 for Chi Square and about 0.015 for SAD. Because the expected values are the same under F as under P, the observed value of Chi Square and SAD depends only on the data, and not on which hypothesis. However, their realized significances DO depend on which hypothesis. In general, a test statistic will have a different realized significance under different hypotheses. In this example, the indications of which cells to interpret are qualitatively the same under the two hypotheses, with P making it quantitatively more clear which they are. I believe these pictures are a small sample of all there were historically, so I would be better advised by hypothesis F. Thus my license to interpret is clear, but what to interpret is less clear.

Hypotheses of dependence

Some scholars have encountered situations in which it is appropriate that some of the boxes in the observed contingency with no observed cases remain empty during simulation. For example, in a study of human behavior, a person was observed smoking a cigarette. During this process, the cigarette was in one of four defined positions: In the ash tray, held in the hand between the thumb and index finger, held in the hand between the index and middle finger, or in the mouth. Observers noted every time the position changed, and summarized their observations in a contingency with rows representing the positions changed *from* and columns representing the positions changed *to*. At any given time, the possible *to* positions depend on the present *from* positions. For example, the smoker has to pick up the cigarette from the ash tray before he can put it in his mouth. Also, the observed data are changes; thus the *to* position must always be different from the *from* position. As a consequence, some of the counts in the boxes of the observed contingency have to be 0. The classical distribution for the Chi Square statistic would be inappropriate for this contingency, even with a very large number of observed changes. An ACTUS2 F or P hypothesis analysis would also be inappropriate, even with only a few observed changes. Here are some example data:

The column labels are:	The row labels are:
Col 1: Ash Tray	Row 1: Ash Tray
Col 2: Thumb and Index Fingers	Row 2: Thumb and Index Fingers
Col 3: Index and Middle Fingers	Row 3: Index and Middle Fingers
Col 4: Mouth	Row 4: Mouth

Counts of movements from the row to the column:

	A	T	I	M
A	0	2	0	0
T	2	0	5	0
I	0	3	0	3
M	0	4	0	0

To start, we will look at an (inappropriate) analysis by ACTUS2 using F-simulation, and then analyze these counts and restrictions to test a hypothesis of dependency that ACTUS2 uses in cases like this.

Expected numbers of observations if rows and columns are independent:

	A	T	I	M	RF
A	0.2	0.9	0.5	0.3	2
T	0.7	3.3	1.8	1.1	7
I	0.6	2.8	1.6	0.9	6
M	0.4	1.9	1.1	0.6	4
CF	2	9	5	3	19

Deviations of observed counts from these expected values:

	A	T	I	M
A	−0.2	1.1	−0.5	−0.3
T	1.3	−3.3	3.2	−1.1
I	−0.6	0.2	−1.6	2.1
M	−0.4	2.1	−1.1	−0.6

F-simulated BIG array:

	A	T	I	M
A	1000	262	1000	1000
T	177	1000	21	1000
I	1000	546	1000	66
M	1000	118	1000	1000

This result suggests that the tendency of the smoker to change from holding the cigarette between thumb and index to holding it between index and middle is strong, with a preference to put it, held that way, in his mouth. These results seem reasonable.

F-simulated SMALL array:

	A	T	I	M
A	807	930	611	715
T	966	31	922	307
I	505	702	196	991
M	683	963	329	512

The failure to ever keep holding the cigarette between the thumb and index finger looks significant, but, of course that box must contain 0 because that change would never be observed as data. Under an appropriate hypothesis, all of the boxes that should continue to contain 0 in the simulated arrays should contain 1000 in the SMALL array, because every simulated array would have a count in such boxes at least as small.

To accommodate cases like this, ACTUS can simulate a so-called R hypothesis of partial dependence. Under the R hypothesis of ACTUS2, you indicate with an R which empty boxes remain empty depending on the row in which they occur. Under the so-called C hypothesis, you indicate such boxes with a C because they remain empty depending on the column in which they occur. In the present example, the R hypothesis is appropriate. A box in the array of observed counts shown below contains an R to indicate that it always contains 0 because, depending on that row, the column of that box is impossible.

	A	T	I	M
A	R	2	0	R
T	2	R	5	0
I	0	3	R	3
M	R	4	0	R

The R hypothesis states that for each row the probabilities of the possible columns are proportional to the number of cases in them. Thus the expected column frequencies are not necessarily the same as the observed column frequencies, as shown in the array below.

R expected values, with expected column frequencies (ECF):

	A	T	I	M	RF
A	0.0	1.3	0.7	0.0	2
T	1.4	0.0	3.5	2.1	2
I	0.9	3.9	0.0	1.3	6
M	0.0	2.6	1.4	0.0	4
CF	2	9	5	3	19
ECF	2.3	7.7	5.6	3.4	

Deviations of observed counts from R expected values:

	A	T	I	M
A	0.0	0.7	−0.7	0.0
T	0.6	0.0	1.5	−2.1
I	−0.9	−0.9	0.0	1.7
M	0.0	1.4	−1.4	0.0

Under the R hypothesis, the impossible boxes remain empty, so their expected value is 0.0, from which the observed value never deviates, as indicated by 0.0 in all the boxes that contain R in the array of observed counts. ACTUS2 used these expected values to calculate an observed value for the Chi Square and SAD statistics. The SAD values calculated from R-simulated arrays were equal to or exceeded the SAD value calculated from the observed counts (11.914), 63 times out of 10 000. The Chi Square values calculated from R-simulated arrays were equal to or exceeded the Chi Square value calculated from the observed counts (9.667), 116 times out of 10000. Both are very significant.

Notice that under these hypotheses of dependency, the expected values are different from the expected values under a hypothesis of independence. Chi Square and SAD statistics are calculated using both the observed counts and their expected values. In this way, the observed values of these statistics depend on hypothesis.

R-simulated SMALL array:

	A	T	I	M
A	1000	852	472	1000
T	845	1000	875	111
I	395	438	1000	975
M	1000	890	241	1000

No counts are clearly small. However, because the whole contingency is very significant, the suggestion that this smoker is unlikely to put the cigarette in his mouth holding it with thumb and index finger may be valid.

R-simulated BIG array:

	A	T	I	M
A	1000	371	1000	1000
T	412	1000	274	1000
I	1000	766	1000	118
M	1000	263	1000	1000

No counts are clearly big. However, because the whole contingency is very significant, the suggestion that this smoker is most likely to put the cigarette in his mouth holding it between index and middle finger may be valid. The number of observed changes in the observed array of counts in this example is quite small. If more observations showed the same tendencies, their significances would be stronger.

Under the R dependent hypothesis, the significances under the F independent hypothesis of the required empty boxes disappear. Compared with the significances under the inappropriate F hypothesis, the significances of the large and small counts among the boxes not required to be empty can change very substantially. Unlike P and F hypotheses of independence, which usually give qualitatively similar results, appropriate use of the R or C hypotheses of partial dependence usually give results that are quite different from the inappropriate use of F or P for the same observed counts.

More than 40 publications have now cited the original ACTUS publications. I have selected a few to give you an idea of the variety of subjects that they have addressed:

Almada *et al.* (1994) Breeding Ecology of *Salaria-Pavo* (a fish)
Amorim and Hawkins (2000) Sounds made by fish
De Amicis and Marchetti (2000) Plant Intercodon dinucleotides
Domingues *et al.* (2007) Molecular evolution of *Coryphoblennius* (fish)
Estabrook, C. B. (1999) Social history of Bristol UK 1660–1780
Estabrook, V. H. (2007) Trauma shown in the bones of Neandertals
Galhardo *et al.* (2008) Effect of substrate on cichlid (fish) welfare
Hawkins and Amorim (2000) Spawning of *Melanogrammus* (haddock)
Marques 2004 Parental care and mate desertion by *Passer* (Sparrows)
Picanco *et al.* (2009) Distribution of whales in Sao Tome and Principe
Raguso and Willis (2002) Visual and olfactory cues used by hawk moths
Ruas and Lechner (1997) Allele frequency in a human population.
Thaker *et al.* (2009) Anti-predator behaviors in male tree lizards
Woldu and Feoli (2001) Shrubland vegetation of Northern Ethiopia
Zambelli *et al.* (2009) Harm to bats from too small forearm bands

11.3   Spreadsheet ACTUS

The purpose of this book is to help you learn how to write spreadsheet macros to take a computational approach to statistical argument, which can free you from the constraints and mysteries of classical statistics, and from dependency on canned programs. However, many scholars encounter the need to analyze sparse contingencies. So as a final example, I show you the complete spreadsheet ACTUS, saved in ACTUS.XLS. Use ACTUS.XLS in your own work, and give it to your colleagues to show them the power and flexibility of a computational approach to statistical argument.

In the course of developing this text, I implemented the two hypotheses of independence of ACTUS2 as an EXCEL macro. ACTUS in macro form has many advantages. Because I now use spreadsheet macros to teach my course on a computational approach to statistical argument, my students are familiar with this form. Most students and other early- or mid- career professionals are familiar with spreadsheets, even if not with macro programming, so that presenting their data for analysis in the form of a spreadsheet does not require much new learning in an unfamiliar environment. Also, it is very easy to give away copies of ACTUS.XLS containing the ACTUS macro ready to run. Most versions of EXCEL running on different computers with different operating systems can open and run the same spreadsheet. This makes the ACTUS.XLS version somewhat JAVA-like in the ease with which you can transfer it from one computer to another.

Design the spreadsheet

Part of designing ACTUS as an EXCEL macro requires deciding where on the spreadsheet ACTUS should read the observed contingency and the chosen hypothesis, and where on the spreadsheet ACTUS should write its results. I decided that ACTUS should read and write on "Sheet1". After ACTUS has written its results, you can rename "Sheet1", giving it a name to help you remember what is on it. If you want to analyze another contingency, rename another worksheet "Sheet1" and enter your counts there. ACTUS reads your chosen hypothesis as F or P from "Cell(1,1)" in the upper left corner. It reads column labels from the cells in row 1, starting with the cell in the second column and continuing one cell at a time; ACTUS will know that all column labels have been read when the next cell contains only "&". It reads the row labels from column 1, starting with the cell in the second row and continuing one cell at a time until the next cell contains only "&". ACTUS then reads your counts in the cells at the intersections of the rows and columns you have labeled. It is a good idea to leave blank the rest of "Sheet1", until after ACTUS writes its results there. I decided to reserve space in memory for an array with up to 12 rows and up to 12 columns. If you have learned some macro programming, you can change these limits. However, arguing with contingencies is very context dependent; if your array gets too big, it may become difficult to interpret correctly. My 2002 publication in *Historical Methods* explains this and gives examples.

Report results

Below the array of counts, ACTUS write the expected values for each box, together with row and column totals, and the grand total. Then it reports the observed value and realized significance of the Chi Square statistic, and of another whole-contingency goodness-of-fit statistic, SAD, sum of the absolute differences between the observed count and the expected count in each box.

SAD differs from Chi Square in that boxes with larger expected values are more likely to contribute relatively more to the value of SAD, and boxes with large absolute differences are likely to contribute relatively less to the value of SAD. Usually their realized significances are similar, with SAD often a little more conservative of the hypothesis of independence.

Below this, ACTUS finally writes two more arrays with the realized significances of the count in each box. The BIG array identifies boxes with observed counts that are too big to be consistent with the hypothesis of independence by reporting the number of simulated data sets (out of 1000, ACTUS simulates 10000 data sets to make its estimates) with counts at least as big as the count observed in that box. Similarly, the SMALL array reports the number of simulated data sets with counts at least as small as the count observed in that box. Examples of ACTUS results were given in the previous section.

How to run ACTUS.XLS

Here are some hints about running ACTUS.XLS. When you first open ACTUS.XLS, it may ask you whether you want to enable macros; yes you do. After you have edited "Sheet1" to enter your hypothesis, row and column labels, and counts in the upper left, save your spreadsheet before running macro ACTUS. To run macro ACTUS bring down the "tools" menu, click on "macros" and, in the menu that pops out, click on "macros" again. This produces a list of macros, in which the only macro is ACTUS; click on "run". The entries in your array of counts must be whole numbers (or blank, which ACTUS will read as 0). In the spreadsheet cells, letters are usually left justified and numbers are usually right justified, so if (for example) you type an *el* for a one or an *oh* for a zero, you can see it right away. If you get a message that says "runtime error 13: type mismatch" it means that you have entered a count that is not a whole number. ACTUS may write its results with inconvenient numbers of decimal places. For the observed values of SAD, CHI, and for the expected values of counts, normally two decimal places are appropriate. For realized significances of CHI and SAD, normally four decimal places are appropriate. The BIG and SMALL tables should have no decimal places. To change the number of decimal places shown in EXCEL cells, highlight the cell (or block of cells); then click on "format", then on "cells". In the box that opens, choose "number" on the left, and on the right scroll up or down to the desired number of decimal places. Even though ACTUS simulates 10000 data sets, on most modern computers this will take less than a minute, unless your table of counts has hundreds of cases. While ACTUS is running, it writes, in row 1 column 16, the number of data sets it has simulated so far. If you have asked ACTUS to analyze a very large number of cases, you can watch this box to see the progress, so not to get too anxious waiting for a few minutes. Remember, every time you edit "Sheet1", you need to save it before you can run macro ACTUS again.

You can use "Save As" to save a copy of the whole ACTUS.XLS workbook in a different location or under a different name. When you do this, you save a copy of your spreadsheets and also the ACTUS macro. This makes it easy to give ACTUS.XLS to your colleagues or students.

11.4   Sub ACTUS

```
Sub ACTUS()
MsgBox " Begin ACTUS"
Dim OK As Boolean              'To return after input errors
Dim HYP As String              'F or P to indicate hypothesis
Dim R, C As Integer            'Index to read/write Rows or Columns
Dim ROWLAB(12) As String       'Row Labels
Dim NR As Byte                 'Number of rows
Dim COLLAB(12) As String       'Column labels
Dim NC As Byte                 'Number of columns
Dim LAB As String              'read next label
Dim COUNTS(12, 12) As Integer  'table of counts
Dim RT(12) As Integer          'Row totals
Dim CT(12) As Integer          'Column totals
Dim GT As Integer              'Grand total
Dim EXPE(12, 12) As Single     'expected values of counts
Dim CHI, SAD As Single         'observed value of CHISQUARE and SAD
statistics
Dim PTAB(2000) As Byte         'permutation table for P
Dim RP(12), CP(12) As Single   'Probabilities of rows and columns for F
Dim BIG(12, 12) As Integer     'Significances of big counts
Dim SMALL(12, 12) As Integer   'Significance of small counts
Dim NS As Integer              'count number of simulations
Dim SCOUNTS(12, 12) As Integer 'simulated counts
Dim I, J As Integer            'Indices for permutation table and SCOUNTS
Dim K As Integer               ' report # simulations
```

```
Dim NL As Integer           'Number left to swap during permutation
Dim X As Single             ' to sample Rnd
Dim HOLD As Byte            'To hold place in PTAB() while swapping
Dim SCHI, SSAD As Single    'Simulated values of CHI and SAD
Dim CHISIG, SADSIG As Integer 'Realized significances of CHI and SAD
Dim SIG As Single           'For reporting CHISIG and SADSIG
'Begin ACTUS instructions
OK = True
HYP = Worksheets("Sheet1").Cells(1, 1)
If Not ((HYP = "P") Or (HYP = "F")) Then
   Worksheets("Sheet1").Cells(1, 16) = "HYP ="
   Worksheets("Sheet1").Cells(1, 17) = HYP
   MsgBox ("Hypothesis in Cell(1,1) must be F or P ")
   OK = False
   End If
If OK Then
   NC = 0
   C = 2
   LAB = Worksheets("Sheet1").Cells(1, C)
   Do Until ((LAB = "") Or Not OK)        'read column labels
      NC = NC + 1
      If NC > 12 Then
         MsgBox ("Number of columns may not exceed 12")
         OK = False
      Else
         COLLAB(NC) = LAB
         C = C + 1
         LAB = Worksheets("Sheet1").Cells(1, C)
         End If
      Loop 'LAB =
   If (NC < 2) Then
      MsgBox ("Number of columns must be at least 2")
      OK = False
      End If ' (NC
   End If 'OK
If OK Then
   NR = 0
   R = 2
   LAB = Worksheets("Sheet1").Cells(R, 1)
```

```
   Do Until ((LAB = "") Or Not OK)              'read row labels
     NR = NR + 1
     If NR > 12 Then
        MsgBox ("Number of rows may not exceed 12")
        OK = False
     Else
        ROWLAB (NR) = LAB
        R = R + 1
        LAB = Worksheets ("Sheet1").Cells (R, 1)
        End If
     Loop 'LAB =
   If (NR < 2) Then
     MsgBox ("Number of rows must be at least 2")
     OK = False
     End If '(NR
   End If 'OK
If OK Then
   For R = 1 To NR
     For C = 1 To NC
        COUNTS (R, C) = Worksheets ("Sheet1").Cells (R + 1, C + 1)
        Next C
     Next R
   GT = 0
   For C = 1 To NC
     CT (C) = 0
     Next C
   For R = 1 To NR 'add up row and column totals
     RT (R) = 0
     For C = 1 To NC
        RT (R) = RT (R) + COUNTS (R, C)
        CT (C) = CT (C) + COUNTS (R, C)
        GT = GT + COUNTS (R, C)
        Next C
     Next R
   If (GT > 2000) And (HYP = "P") Then
     Worksheets ("Sheet1").Cells (2, 16) = "GT ="
     Worksheets ("Sheet1").Cells (2, 17) = GT
     MsgBox ("Number of cases may not exceed 2000 for hypothesis P")
     OK = False
```

```
      End If ` (GT
    End If `OK
If OK Then `Execute the rest of the program
For R = 1 To NR
    For C = 1 To NC
      If CT(C) > RT(R) Then `avoid overflow with very large counts
        EXPE(R, C) = (CT(C) / GT) * RT(R)
      Else
        EXPE(R, C) = (RT(R) / GT) * CT(C)
        End If
      Next C
    Next R
`Write Expected table to worksheet
Worksheets("Sheet1").Cells(NR + 3, 1) = "Expected"
For R = 1 To NR
    Worksheets("Sheet1").Cells(NR + 4 + R, 1) = ROWLAB(R)
    Next R
Worksheets("Sheet1").Cells(NR + 4 + NR + 1, 1) = "Col Total"
For C = 1 To NC
    Worksheets("Sheet1").Cells(NR + 4, C + 1) = COLLAB(C)
    Next C
Worksheets("Sheet1").Cells(NR + 4, NC + 2) = "Row Total"
For R = 1 To NR
    For C = 1 To NC
      Worksheets("Sheet1").Cells(NR + 4 + R, C + 1) = EXPE(R, C)
      Next C
    Worksheets("Sheet1").Cells(NR + 4 + R, NC + 2) = RT(R)
    Next R
For C = 1 To NC
    Worksheets("Sheet1").Cells(NR + 4 + NR + 1, C + 1) = CT(C)
    Worksheets("Sheet1").Cells(NR + 4 + NR + 1, NC + 2) = GT
    Next C
`Calculate observed values for CHI and SAD
CHI = 0
SAD = 0
For R = 1 To NR
    For C = 1 To NC
    If EXPE(R, C) <> 0 Then
      X = (COUNTS(R, C) - EXPE(R, C)) * (COUNTS(R, C) - EXPE(R, C))
```

```
        X = X / EXPE(R,C)
        CHI = CHI + X
        End If
     If COUNTS(R, C) - EXPE(R, C) > 0 Then
        SAD = SAD + COUNTS(R, C) - EXPE(R, C)
        Else
        SAD = SAD + EXPE(R, C) - COUNTS(R, C)
        End If
     Next C
  Next R
  If HYP = "P" Then 'Make PTAB
     I = 0
     For R = 1 To NR
        For J = 1 To RT(R)
           I = I + 1
           PTAB(I) = R
           Next J
        Next R
     Else 'which means End the If part
  'Initialize RP() and CP()
     For R = 1 To NR
        RP(R) = RT(R) / GT
        Next R
     For R = 2 To NR
        RP(R) = RP(R) + RP(R - 1)
        Next R
     For C = 1 To NC
        CP(C) = CT(C) / GT
        Next C
     For C = 2 To NC
        CP(C) = CP(C) + CP(C - 1)
        Next C
     End If 'which means End the Else part
  'Initialize BIG() and SMALL()
  For R = 1 To NR
     For C = 1 To NC
        BIG(R, C) = 0
        SMALL(R, C) = 0
        Next C
```

```
    Next R
CHISIG = 0
SADSIG = 0
Randomize
K = 0
Worksheets("Sheet1").Cells(1, 15) = "# Sims ="
For NS = 1 To 10000    'Simulate 10000 data sets
   For R = 1 To NR    'initialize SCOUNTS()
      For C = 1 To NC
         SCOUNTS(R, C) = 0
         Next C
      Next R
   If HYP = "P" Then
      'Permute PTAB
      NL = GT
      For I = 1 To GT - 1
         X = Rnd * NL
         J = 1
         Do Until J > X
            J = J + 1
            Loop
         If J <> NL Then 'switch contents of PTAB(J) and PTAB(NL)
            HOLD = PTAB(J)
            PTAB(J) = PTAB(NL)
            PTAB(NL) = HOLD
            End If
         NL = NL - 1
         Next I
      'Load SCOUNTS() under P
      I = 0
      For C = 1 To NC
         For J = 1 To CT(C)
            I = I + 1
            SCOUNTS(PTAB(I), C) = SCOUNTS(PTAB(I), C) + 1
            Next J
         Next C
      Else 'If HYP.. It is silly, but in VB you end the If with Else
            'and you end the Else with End If
      'Load SCOUNTS() under F
```

```
For I = 1 To GT
   X = Rnd
   R = 1
   Do While X > RP(R)
      R = R + 1
      Loop
   X = Rnd
   C = 1
   Do While X > CP(C)
      C = C + 1
      Loop
   SCOUNTS(R, C) = SCOUNTS(R, C) + 1
   Next I
   End If
'Calculate simulated values for CHI and SAD
SCHI = 0
SSAD = 0
For R = 1 To NR
   For C = 1 To NC
   If EXPE(R, C) <> 0 Then
      X = (SCOUNTS(R,C) - EXPE(R,C)) * (SCOUNTS(R,C) - EXPE(R,C))
      X = X / EXPE(R,C)
      SCHI = SCHI + X
      End If
   If SCOUNTS(R, C) - EXPE(R, C) > 0 Then
      SSAD = SSAD + SCOUNTS(R, C) - EXPE(R, C)
      Else
      SSAD = SSAD + EXPE(R, C) - SCOUNTS(R, C)
      End If
   Next C
Next R
If SSAD >= SAD Then
   SADSIG = SADSIG + 1
   End If
If SCHI >= CHI Then
   CHISIG = CHISIG + 1
   End If
'Load BIG and SMALL
For R = 1 To NR
```

```
    For C = 1 To NC
      If COUNTS (R, C) >= SCOUNTS (R, C) Then
        SMALL (R, C) = SMALL (R, C) + 1
        End If
      If COUNTS (R, C) <= SCOUNTS (R, C) Then
        BIG (R, C) = BIG (R, C) + 1
        End If
      Next C
    Next R
  K = K + 1
  If K = 500 Then
    K = 0
    Worksheets ("Sheet1") .Cells (1, 16) = NS
    Randomize
    End If
  Next NS
'report SAD and CHI values and realized significance
Worksheets ("Sheet1") .Cells (2 * NR + 7, 1) = HYP
Worksheets ("Sheet1") .Cells (2 * NR + 7, 2) = "SAD ="
Worksheets ("Sheet1") .Cells (2 * NR + 7, 3) = SAD
Worksheets ("Sheet1") .Cells (2 * NR + 7, 5) = "CHI ="
Worksheets ("Sheet1") .Cells (2 * NR + 7, 6) = CHI
Worksheets ("Sheet1") .Cells (2 * NR + 8, 2) = "SAD Sig ="
SIG = SADSIG / 10000
Worksheets ("Sheet1") .Cells (2 * NR + 8, 3) = SIG
Worksheets ("Sheet1") .Cells (2 * NR + 8, 5) = "CHI Sig ="
SIG = CHISIG / 10000
Worksheets ("Sheet1") .Cells (2 * NR + 8, 6) = SIG
Worksheets ("Sheet1") .Cells (2 * NR + 11, 1) = "BIG"
Worksheets ("Sheet1") .Cells (2 * NR + 12, 1) = HYP
  For R = 1 To NR
    Worksheets ("Sheet1") .Cells (2 * NR + 12 + R, 1) = ROWLAB (R)
    Next R
  For C = 1 To NC
    Worksheets ("Sheet1") .Cells (2 * NR + 12, C + 1) = COLLAB (C)
    Next C
  For R = 1 To NR
    For C = 1 To NC
      K = Round (BIG (R, C) / 10)
```

```
            Worksheets("Sheet1").Cells(2 * NR + 12 + R, C + 1) = K
            Next C
        Next R
    Worksheets("Sheet1").Cells(3 * NR + 15, 1) = "SMALL"
    Worksheets("Sheet1").Cells(3 * NR + 16, 1) = HYP
    For R = 1 To NR
        Worksheets("Sheet1").Cells(3 * NR + 16 + R, 1) = ROWLAB(R)
        Next R
    For C = 1 To NC
        Worksheets("Sheet1").Cells(3 * NR + 16, C + 1) = COLLAB(C)
        Next C
    For R = 1 To NR
        For C = 1 To NC
            K = Round(SMALL(R, C) / 10)
            Worksheets("Sheet1").Cells(3 * NR + 16 + R, C + 1) = K
            Next C
        Next R
End If 'OK to execute the rest of the program
If Not OK Then 'input errors because counts are not on "Sheet1" ?
    MsgBox ("Is your contingency table in the upper left of Sheet1?")
    End If
MsgBox ("End ACTUS")
End Sub
```

References

Almada, V. C., Goncalves, E. J., Santos, A. J. and Baptista, C. (1994) Breeding ecology and nest aggregations in a population of *Salaria-Pavo* (Pisces, Blenniidae) in an area where nest sites are very scarce. *Journal of Fish Biology*. **45**: 819–830.

Amorim, M. C. P. and Hawkins, A. D. (2000) Growling for food: acoustic emissions during competitive feeding of the streaked gurnard. *Journal of Fish Biology*. **57**: 895–907.

De Amicis, F. and Marchetti, S. (2000) Intercodon dinucleotides affect codon choice in plant genes. *Nucleic Acids Research*. **28**: 3339–3345.

Domingues, V. S., Faria, C., Stefanni, S., Santos, R. S., Brito, A. and Almada, V. C. (2007) Genetic divergence in the Atlantic-Mediterranean Montagu's blenny, Coryphoblennius galerita (Linnaeus 1758) revealed by molecular and morphological characters. *Molecular Ecology*. **16**: 3592–3605.

Efron, B. (1979) Computers and the theory of statistics – thinking the unthinkable. *Siam Review*. **21**: 460–480.

Efron, B. and Tibshirani, R. (1986) Boot strap methods for confidence intervals and other measures of statistical accuracy. *Statistical Science*. **1**: 54–77.

Estabrook, C. B. and Estabrook, G. F. (1989) ACTUS: a solution to the problem of small samples in the analysis of 2-way contingency-tables. *Historical Methods*. **22**: 5–8.

Estabrook, C. B. (1999) *Urbane and Rustic England: Cultural Ties and Social Spheres in the Provinces 1660–1780 (Politics, Culture & Society in Early Modern Britain)*. Manchester, UK: Manchester University Press.

Estabrook, G. F. and Jespersen, D. C. (1974) Strategy for a predator encountering a model-mimic system. *American Naturalist*. **108**: 443–457.

Estabrook, G. F. (2002) Two hypotheses of independence for the recognition of qualitative co-occurrences in small amounts of data. *Historical Methods*. **35**: 21–31.

Estabrook, V. H. (2007) Is trauma at Krapina like all other Neandertal trauma? A statistical comparison of trauma patterns in Neandertal skeletal remains. *Periodicum Biologorum*. **109**: 393–400.

Feller, W. (1957) *An Introduction to Probability Theory and Its Applications, Volumes I and II*. New York: John Wiley and Sons, Inc.

Galhardo, L., Correia, J. and Oliveira, R. F. (2008) The effect of substrate availability on behavioural and physiological indicators of welfare in the African cichlid (*Oreochromis mossambicus*). *Animal Welfare*. **17**: 239–254.

Gilinsky, N. L. (1986) Was there 26-Myr periodicity of extinctions? *Nature*. **321**: 533–534.

Gorchov, D. L. and Estabrook, G. F. (1987) A test of several hypotheses for the determination of seed number in *Amelanchier arborea*, using simulated probability-distributions to evaluate data. *American Journal of Botany*. **74**: 1893–1897.

Hawkins, A. D. and Amorim, M. C. P. (2000) Spawning sounds of the male haddock, *Melanogrammus aeglefinus*. *Environmental Biology of Fishes*. **59**: 29–41.

Hoffman, A. (1986) Was there 26-Myr periodicity of extinctions – reply. *Nature*. **321**: 535–536.

Hoogendyk, C. G. and Estabrook, G. F. (1984) The consequences of earlier reproduction in declining populations. *Mathematical Biosciences*. **71**: 217–235.

Kemeny, J. G. (1964) *Finite Mathematical Structures*. New York: Prentice Hall.

Kitchell, J. A. and Estabrook, G. (1986) Was there 26-Myr periodicity of extinctions? *Nature*. **321**: 534–535.

Kitchell, J. A., Estabrook, G. F. and Macleod, N. (1987) Testing for equality of rates of evolution. *Paleobiology*. **13**: 272–285.

Marques, P. A. M. (2004) Parental care during incubation in Spanish Sparrows Passer hispaniolensis: sex roles and effect of male mate desertion. *Bird Study*. **51**: 185–188.

Mertz, D. B. (1971) Mathematical demography of California Condor population. *American Naturalist*. **105**: 437.

Picanco, C., Carvalho, I. and Brito, C. (2009) Occurrence and distribution of cetaceans in Sao Tome and Principe tropical archipelago and their relation to environmental variables. *Journal of the Marine Biological Association of the United Kingdom*. **89**: 1071–1076.

Raguso, R. A. and Willis, M. A. (2002) Synergy between visual and olfactory cues in nectar feeding by naive hawkmoths, *Manduca sexta*. *Animal Behaviour*. **64**: 685–695.

Raup, D. M. and Sepkoski, J. J. (1984a) Periodicity of extinctions in the geologic past. *Proceedings of the National Academy of Sciences of the United States of America-Biological Sciences*. **81**: 801–805.

Raup, D. M. and Sepkoski, J. J. (1984b) Publishing chronology. *Nature*. **309**: 300–300.

Ruas, J. L. and Lechner, M. C. (1997) Allele frequency of CYP2C19 in a Portuguese population. *Pharmacogenetics*. **7**: 333–335.

Schildt, H. (1986) *Advanced Turbo Pascal*. New York: McGraw Hill.

Sepkoski, J. J. and Raup, D. M. (1986) Was there 26-Myr periodicity of extinctions? *Nature*. **321**: 533.

Stutz, A. J. and Estabrook, G. F. (2002) A computationally intensive statistical technique for analyzing interassemblage variability in lithic type frequency distributions, with an application to the Epipaleolithic of the Levant. *Journal of Human Evolution*. **42**: A35.

Thaker, M., Lima, S. L. and Hews, D. K. (2009) Acute corticosterone elevation enhances antipredator behaviors in male tree lizard morphs. *Hormones and Behavior*. **56**: 51–57.

Woldu, Z. and Feoli, E. (2001) The shrubland vegetation of Adwa, Northern Ethiopia. In *Biodiversity Research in the Horn of Africa Region*. Friis, I. and Ryding, O. (eds.), pp. 319–333.

Zambelli, N., Moretti, M., Mattei-Roesli, M. and Bontadina, F. (2009) Negative consequences of forearm bands that are too small for bats. *Acta Chiropterologica*. **11**: 216–219.

Index

Printed in the United States
by Baker & Taylor Publisher Services